Experimental Leukemia and Mammary Cancer

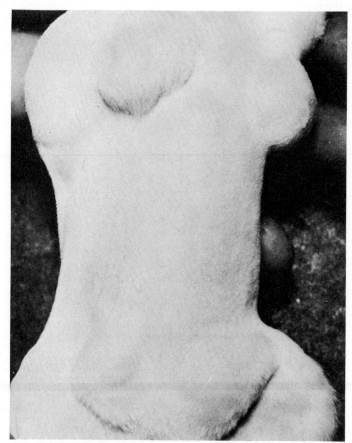

Mammary cancers in pectoral and inguinal regions of a young adult
female Sprague-Dawley rat elicited by a single feeding of
20 mg of 7,12-dimethylbenz[a]anthracene 50 days previously.

Experimental Leukemia and Mammary Cancer

Induction, Prevention, Cure

Charles Brenton Huggins, M.D.

The University of Chicago Press

Chicago and London

CHARLES BRENTON HUGGINS has been a member of the
faculty of the University of Chicago since 1927.
From 1951 to 1969 he was director of the Ben May
Laboratory for Cancer Research and he has been the
William B. Ogden Distinguished Service Professor
since 1962. In 1966 he won the Nobel Prize in
medicine and physiology for his work on carcinoma
of the prostate.

The University of Chicago Press, Chicago 60637
The University of Chicago Press, Ltd., London

83 82 81 80 79   5 4 3 2 1

Library of Congress Cataloging in Publication Data

Huggins, Charles, 1901–
    Experimental leukemia and mammary cancer.

    Bibliography: p.
    Includes index.
    1. Oncology, Experimental. 2. Mammary glands—
Cancer—Research. 3. Leukemia—Research.
4. Rats—Physiology. 5. Mice—Physiology.
I. Title.
RC267.H79   616.1′55′027   78-25790
ISBN 0-226-35860-7

To Margaret Wellman Huggins

Contents

Preface

This volume is a commonplace book describing our ways to induce, to prevent, and to eradicate leukemia and mammary cancer in rodents. The methods were devised during twenty years of uninterrupted investigation in fine laboratories at the University of Chicago. It is the "Chicago catechism."

One works along at the lab bench without haste and without rest. Time has no meaning; every day something will be done, something will be found out. It is total commitment to the task at hand. It requires Spartan self-discipline. These are happy days, one following another, hopefully without end, so great is the delight of discovery.

Always, the students are here—not many of them because, with Paul Ehrlich, I believe that great creative things do not emerge with too many pigeons flying about the room. The students are necessary and a joy. Discussion is helpful in originating new ideas and in bringing out the strength and weakness of the protocol. Both the eye and ear are useful in the design of the great plan and, at the end of the experiment, in admiration of elegant results. The student provides zing; he has great self-confidence and the energy of youth and, for him, always there is the carrot, never the stick.

In the biological sciences research is the "quiet art," a cottage industry done in the *stoa*, where one can work with the students in serenity ten or more hours a day with an abiding faith that the world's most vexatious medical problems here can be solved and very soon.

Science is not cold and unfeeling. In scientific investigation one becomes emotionally contained in his problem. Head, heart, and hand, the three *H*'s of experimentation, all are involved in innovation in the medical sciences and the combination enables us to recognize a good problem that can be solved. Science is ruled by idea and technique, which are welded to form a wheel that revolves and gains momentum. Activity arouses idea, which in turn begets method. With blood on my hands I can discover; seated at my desk I have no chance. This is the philosophy of activism, which governs science.

In science one always strives for simplicity, which is the elegance of proof: Simplex sigillium veri.

The work of our laboratory described in this volume was done in collaboration with an outstanding group of young scientists. I am much indebted to my coworkers:

Delbert M. Bergenstal
Colin Bird
Filomena P. Brillantes
Giuliano Briziarelli
Alan K. Burnett
Anne Stack Cleveland
Heinz Dannenberg
Thomas L. Dao
Thomas Franklin Deuel
George C. Fareed
Elizabeth Ford
Ryo Fukunishi
Lorraine Grand
Ronald G. Harvey
Elwood V. Jensen
Ichiro Kuwahara
Klaus Mainzer
Richard C. Moon
Sotokichi Morii

Peter Vincent Moulder
Hisao Oka
Ryohei Okamoto
John Pataki
A. H. Reddi
E. Douglas Rees
Anna Maria Russo
Paul E. Schurr
Taketoshi Sugiyama
Harold G. Sutton, Jr.
Katherine L. Sydnor
Paul Talalay
Norifumi Ueda
Kunio Uematsu
H. G. Williams-Ashman
Solomon Wiseman
N. C. Yang
Hiroshi Yoshida

Acknowledgments

This work was supported by grants from the American Cancer Society, the Jane Coffin Childs Memorial Fund for Medical Research, and by grant number 11603-09 awarded by the National Cancer Institute, Department of Health, Education, and Welfare.

This book could not have been written without the splendid secretarial assistance of Mrs. Louise Gustafson Alexander.

CHARLES BRENTON HUGGINS

The Ben May Laboratory for Cancer Research
The University of Chicago

Abbreviations and Trivial Names

AAF	2-acetylaminofluorene
AAT	o-aminoazotoluene
ACTH	corticotrophin
AH	adenohypophysis
AS	aminostilbene
asp	asparaginase
BA	benz[a]anthracene
BGH	bovine growth hormone
BHK	baby hamster kidney
BP	benzo[a]pyrene
C1628	1-{2-(p-[α(p-methoxyphenyl)-β-nitrostyryl]phenoxy)ethyl} pyrrolidine
Chloramiphene	1-(p-β-diethylaminoethoxyphenyl)-1,2-diphenyl-2-chloroethylene
Clomiphene	see Chloramiphene
CML	chronic myelogenous leukemia
ConA	concanavalin A
Cyclic AMP	cyclic adenosine 3′, 5′-monophosphate
DAB	dimethylaminoazobenzene
DBA	dibenz[a,h]anthracene
DEBA	diethylbenz[a]anthracene
DES	see diethylstilbestrol
Diethylstilbestrol	α,α′-diethylstilbenediol
DMAS	dimethylaminostilbene
DMBA	7,12-dimethylbenz[a]anthracene
DMSO	dimethylsulfoxide
DOPA	dihydroxyphenylalanine
DNA	deoxyribonucleic acid
Estradiol	estra-1,3,5(10)-triene-3, 17β-diol
Estriol	estra-1,3,5(10)-triene-3, 16α,17β-triol
Estrone	estra-1,3,5(10)-trien-3-ol-17-one
Et	ethyl
FAD	flavine-adenine dinucleotide

GlcNAc	N-acetylglucosamine
HAN	hyperplastic alveolar nodule
Hb	hemoglobin
His	histidine
Hypox	hypophysectomized
LD_{50}	dosage causing death of half of a series of animals
LDH	lactic dehydrogenase (EC 1.1.1.27)
L-E	Long-Evans
$Leuk_{50}$	day on which leukemia is detected in half of a series of animals
LH	luteinizing hormone
MBA	monomethyl-substituted BA
MC	methylcholanthrene
MDH	malic dehydrogenase (EC 1.1.1.37)
Me	methyl
Me-DAB	dimethylaminoazobenzene
Me-MAB	monomethylaminoazobenzene
MR	menadione reductase (EC 1.6.99.2)
MTV	mammary tumor virus
NAD	nicotinamide-adenine dinucleotide
NADP	nicotinamide-adenine dinucleotide phosphate
Nafoxidine	1-{2-[p-(3,4-dihydro-6-methoxy-2-phenyl-1-naphthyl)phenoxy]ethyl}pyrrolidine
Ovariex	ovariectomized
PAS	periodic acid-Schiff reagents
PEP	polyestradiol phosphate
PHA	phytohemagglutinin
PIF	prolactin inhibitory factor
r	Roentgen units
RNA	ribonucleic acid
RSV	Rous sarcoma virus
SCL	stem-cell leukemia
S-D	Sprague-Dawley
Sudan III	1-(p-phenylazo-phenylazo)-2-naphthol
SV40	simian virus 40
Tace	tris(p-methoxyphenyl)chloroethylene
Tamoxifen	1-(p-β-dimethylaminoethoxyphenyl)-1, 2-diphenylbut-1-ene
TdR	thymidine
TMBA	trimethylbenz[a]anthracene
U-11100A	*see* Nafoxidine

The Cancer Cell

Of all the diseases of man, cancer is the most singular and the most dread. Cancer is a catastrophic disturbance of growth in its host and if it is not checked, man is consumed by his own flesh. The outstanding property of the cancer cell is abnormal and unrestrained growth. Cell growth in active cancers is unregulated but not uncontrollable. Cancer is not a growth of anarchic cells; laws control the survival of the cancer cell and these it must obey. Much is known about cancers, their causes and characteristics, their prevention, the restraint and cure of many cancers by hormonal methods. These matters are dealt with in the present volume from an experimenter's viewpoint.

Cancers have distinctive attributes—all unfavorable and destructive of the host's economy. These common characteristics of cancer include:

i. Infiltration of neighboring tissues with obstruction of vital passages.

ii. Metastasis to distant sites where colonization takes place, destroying and replacing essential physiologic activities such as the formation of blood and antibodies resulting in anemia and weakening of defenses against infection.

iii. An increase in size of cancers which can surpass the formation of accompanying blood vessels. In this way faulty angiogenesis causes the surface of cancers to erode and ulcerate with resultant hemorrhage and secondary infection.

iv. A decrease of appetite, which leads to malnutrition and cachexia. Afflicted with anorexia, the patient starves despite the ready availability of nutritious foods in the kitchen. Notwithstanding a strong will and a compelling incentive to remain alive, the patient without appetite cannot eat. Yet the appetite is restored rapidly after suppression of the cancer. For example, following hormonal control of widespread cancer of the prostate one sees a ravenous appetite develop in an emaciated man within several hours.

Cancer is a special sort of reaction to nonspecific injury. The result is a cell with a false genetic code, a modification of its surface, a decrease of special functions characteristic of its normal cell of origin, and a propensity for exuberant growth.

It would appear that the fundamental lesions in the cancer cell are special and particular alterations of the genome with multiple, consistent, and nonrandom abnormalities in the chromosomes. The abnormalities of the chromosomes are accompanied by a characteristic alteration of the cell surface, which has profound significance for cell growth. The specific injury to the genes can arise from a multitude of causes—just as you can hurt your finger in a thousand ways. Certain agents, for example, boiling water, can cause cancer but rarely do so. Other agents are highly effective in producing cancer and these are designated *carcinogens*.

Specific Changes in Chromosomes: The Karyotype

In an hypothesis of the essential nature of the cancer cell Boveri 1929 stated: "the essence of my theory is not the abnormal mitoses but a *certain abnormal-chromatin complex, no matter how it arises*. Every process which brings about this chromatin condition would lead to a malignant tumor."

Techniques perfected in the last twenty years have made it possible to examine in detail the chromosomes of many species in samples of readily obtainable cells such as leukocytes, tumor cells, and fibroblasts. The karyotype is a systematic array of the cell's chromosomes (fig. 1.1), which makes possible an analysis of the number, form, size, and position of the centromere and the intrachromosomal bands. Three techniques are employed in karyotypic analysis; incubation of the cells in a tissue culture medium; treatment with colchicine, a plant alkaloid that arrests cell division at the stage (metaphase) when the individual chromosomes are most widely separated; and immersion of such preparations in a dilute salt solution, which causes the chromosomes to swell. Tigerlike stripes and bands become apparent when the chromosomes are stained with certain dyes or fluorescent compounds.

The regular appearance of abnormal chromosomes in neoplastic disease supports the hypothesis that alterations in the genome are involved in the transformation of normal cells into malignant ones. Karyotypic analysis of the number and shape of chromosomes in leukemic cells in man (Nowell and Hungerford 1960) and mouse (Stich 1960) revealed consistent nonrandom anomalies in cancer cells. It is certain that specific chromosomal alterations occur frequently in neoplastic cells.

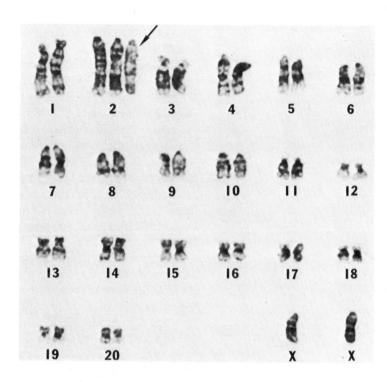

Fig. 1.1. Karyotype of 7,8,12-TMBA-induced erythroleukemia (rat) with no. 2 trisomy. The chromosome numbering system is presented.

How do the characteristic chromosomal changes influence the metabolism, growth rate, and the surface properties of a cancer cell?

The karyotypic aberrations are of three types, deletion, translocation, and trisomy, which is defined as a triploid chromosome in an otherwise diploid set.

Human Malignant Cells. Nonrandom chromosomal aberrations have been found in chromosome nos. 9, 14, and 22 in human cancer cells. In a classic paper on human malignant disease Nowell and Hungerford 1960 first identified a characteristic abnormality, namely, one of the chromosomes in the leukemic cells was unusually small. The observations were made in karyotype studies of a patient afflicted with chronic myelogenous leukemia (CML). An identical chromosome aberration was found in 9 of 10 patients with CML; one of the 4 smallest acrocentric chromosomes in the leukemic cells was greatly reduced in size because of the loss of half of its longer arm; the abnormal chromosome was designated the Ph^1 chromosome. Nowell and Hungerford 1961 state: "The findings demonstrate a specific consistent, chromosome change associated with a particular human neoplasm and suggest that it is the chromosomal change that confers on the leukocytes their neoplastic character."

Rowley 1973 studied chromosomes of leukemic cells of patients with CML by means of quinaquine fluorescence and Giemsa staining. The Ph[1] chromosome represents a deletion of the long arm of one of the paired chromosomes no. 22 (22q−). An unsuspected abnormality in all the leukemic cells was detected by the new staining techniques—it consisted of the addition of dully fluorescing material to the end of the long arm of one chromosome, no. 9 (9q+). The amount of additional material is equal to the amount missing from the Ph[1] (22q−) chromosome; the equal amounts suggest a translocation between the long arm of 22 and the long arm of 9, producing the 9q+ chromosome.

A consistent structural abnormality of chromosome no. 14, an extra band at the end of the long arm, has been found in African Burkitt lymphomas and other types of human malignant lymphoma (Manolov and Manolova 1972; Fukuhara, Shirakawa, and Uchino 1976).

Mark 1973 studied chromosomes in 10 human meningiomas; in each case there was a loss of one chromosome no. 22 in the neoplastic cells.

Mouse Leukemia. Stich 1960 found consistent abnormal chromosomes in experimentally produced lymphomas in mice. One or two subcutaneous injections of 7,12-dimethylbenz[*a*]-anthracene (7,12-DMBA) in Swiss mice resulted in lymphosarcomas in half of the group; 15 of 16 lymphosarcomas of the thymus contained neoplastic cells with 41 chromosomes compared with a modal number of 40 in the normal counterparts. A single small chromosome resembling the Y chromosome in size and shape was observed in the cells of many of the lymphosarcomas. It would appear that the small abnormal chromosome arose from a chromosomal deletion.

Experimental Erythroleukemia in Rat. The experimental leukemias of rats are of special interest since leukemia rarely arises spontaneously in this species but can be induced readily and rapidly by multiple doses of 7,12-DMBA or 7,8,12-TMBA. Repeated doses of these hydrocarbons under stated conditions (p. 119) regularly result in a high incidence (80%–95%) of leukemia in Long-Evans rats and chromosomes from spleen and marrow cells can be prepared readily for cytologic study. Also the morphology of rat chromosomes is such that many of them can be identified individually. Distinctive chromosomal aberrations are frequently observed in the leukemia cells; members of the nos. 1 and 2 chromosome pairs are especially vulnerable to both initial damage and terminal aberration of the chromosomal apparatus.

Sugiyama, Kurita, and Nishizuka 1967 found that many erythroleukemia cells had consistent structural abnormalities of the longest telocentric chromosomes. Among 23 leukemia rats examined, 10 had trisomy of chromosome no. 1 or 2 (fig. 1.1). Although the typical trisomy of chromosome 1 was predominant, some rats had a leukemia cell line characterized by the presence of one no. 1 normal chromosome together with one very long metacentric marker chromosome composed of two no. 1 chromosomes fused together. It was evident that the fused chromosomes are essentially a trisomy of no. 1 chromosome of translocation type. Sugiyama 1971b indicated that the no. 1 chromosome of the rat differs from many other chromosomes in the specific vulnerability of two of its regions, respectively, at regions .29 and .53 of the total length from the centromere; these regions are highly susceptible to the chromosome-damaging action of 7,12-DMBA, especially in late interphase or prophase.

The early stages of carcinogen-induced chromosomal damage have been described by Rees, Majumbar, and Shuck 1970. Twenty-four hours after a single intravenous injection of 7,12-DMBA or 7,8,12-TMBA, about half of the metaphase cells in the marrow have chromosomes with breaks and gaps. Although breaks were inflicted on chromosomes of various sizes and shapes, these aberrations were selective and nonrandom in that members of the no. 1 and no. 2 chromosome pairs were involved to an extent greater than expected on the basis of their size and number. Distinctive karyotypic aberrations involving the no. 2 chromosome were observed in half of the leukemic rats, whereas these abnormalities were not seen in nonleukemic 7,12-DMBA-treated rats.

Karyotypic Changes in Experimental Sarcomas. The sarcomas of fibroblasts induced in albino rat by Rous Sarcoma Virus or by 7,12-DMBA are histologically identical but are characterized by distinctive chromosome patterns (Mitelman and Levan 1972; Mitelman et al. 1972). In the rat the RSV-induced sarcomas exhibit one of the most striking nonrandom patterns ever observed; it involves a characteristic three-stage karyotypic evolution. Chromosome analysis of 12 primary 7,12-DMBA-induced sarcomas in the same inbred rat strain used for RSV studies revealed a completely different chromosome pattern. Among these sarcomas were 10 tumors in which trisomy of the longest terminal chromosome (no. 1) was the first characteristic feature, the second being trisomy of one m chromosome. The chromosomes most often involved in the evolution of the RSV tumors were participating only exceptionally in the variation of the 7,12-DMBA leukemias and sarcomas.

Detection of Chemical Mutagens

Ames et al. 1973 devised ingenious methods for detecting mutagenic chemicals using bacteria as sensitive indicators of damage to DNA. Certain substances, including some chemical carcinogens, induced new mutations in tester strains of *Salmonella* mutants whereas other carcinogenic compounds failed to do so unless they were "activated" (Ames, Lee, and Durston 1973); the activated forms were good mutagens. Some compounds produce frameshifts and some cause base pair substitutions in DNA. The activated compounds were generated by adding hepatic microsomes containing cytochrome P450 monoxygenase enzymes (p. 147) requiring NADPH and O_2 for their activity.

In the Ames assay, liver microsomes are added to the test compounds; the procedure assays the number of revertant colonies developed by the test chemical in a set of histidine-requiring (his⁻) bacterial strains. A mutagen produces a new "reverse mutation" in the Ames test.

In brief, specially selected strains of (his⁻) *Salmonella typhimurium* are seeded as a lawn on a petri plate containing the appropriate culture medium. A drop of test chemical is placed in the center of the plate. If the chemical is a mutagen, a reversion to prototype will occur in an occasional bacterium, which becomes (his⁺), permitting it to grow. Therefore, a ring of colonies surrounding the test chemical indicates that it is mutagenic.

To develop a test with broad sensitivity Ames screened a large number of *Salmonella typhimurium* mutants, which were (his⁻) with a variety of mutagens. The tester strains were chosen from these to detect a spectrum of types of mutagens: those that cause base pair substitutions or cause insertions or deletions of one or two base pairs (frameshift mutations).

In general mutations are reverted most often by the same kind of alteration of the DNA that occurred with the primary mutation. Base pair substitutions are corrected by a second base pair substitution at the primary site, whereas frameshift mutations are compensated for by a second frameshift mutation nearby. Ames found that many carcinogenic polycyclic hydrocarbons are exceedingly powerful frameshift mutagens. These mutagens presumably intercalate into DNA and then react with it.

McCann et al. 1975 tested about 300 chemical compounds for mutagenicity in the *Salmonella* microsome test. A high correlation between carcinogenicity and mutagenicity was found: 90% (156/174) of the carcinogens were mutagenic but 12% (13/108) of noncarcinogens also caused mutations.

The Ames procedure is an informative test of mutagenicity. It is a valuable procedure in cancer research but bacterial DNA lacks specificity for a categorical identification of a chemical carcinogen.

All carcinogens cause mutations; not all mutagenic agents cause cancer.

Glycolysis

The work of Otto Warburg (1883–1970) is characterized by incredible originality, sweep, and scope (Warburg 1948*a, b*). In the study of biological oxidations, Warburg stands in rank with Lavoisier and Pasteur. Much of the methodology of the new biochemistry originated with Warburg. The new methods include: *i*, use of tissue slices in metabolic experiments; *ii*, micromanometric methods indicating respiration and lactate formation (glycolysis); *iii*, spectrophotometry using the photoelectric cell and monochromatic light with measurement of the 340 nm absorption band of reduced pyridine nucleotides; *iv*, isolation and crystallization of pure respiratory and glycolytic enzymes from yeasts and cancers; and *v*, discovery of glycolysis of cancer cells.

Whereas a large number of normal tissues and cancers produce lactic acid from glucose rapidly in the absence of O_2, only tissue slices of cancers and very few normal tissues show an appreciable ability to glycolyse in the presence of O_2. Concerning cancer, Warburg 1930 stated:

Glycolysis is a property of all (malignant) tumours and very different types of tumour agree quantitatively as regards glycolysis to a considerable extent. Moreover this agreement is independent of variations in the original normal tissue, cause, origin or species of animal. The only exceptions to this statement are a few spontaneous tumours of the mouse which do not appear to bring about glycolysis under aerobic conditions.

The first independent experiments of Warburg, done in the Zoological Station in Naples, were concerned with the metabolic changes in ova after fertilization. Warburg 1910 discovered that "If the egg of the sea urchin is fertilized, the oxygen capacity increases in a short time to a marked extent—about sixfold."

The studies on sea urchin eggs led to an investigation of malignant cells: Is oxygen consumption in cancer cells similar to the changes in respiration in the ovum of the sea urchin after it has been fertilized? Does the metabolism of cancer cells differ qualitatively from that of normal tissues?

Warburg, Posener, and Negelein 1924 measured the rates of respiration of the transplantable Flexner-Jobling rat carcinoma using the tissue slice technique and manometry developed for this purpose. The results were clear-cut. First, the rate of oxygen consumption of the cancer cells did not differ from that of a variety of normal cells. Second, cancer cells readily form lactate from glucose to an extent that far exceeds the rates of liver, kidney, pancreas, thyroid, and submaxillary gland. Third, a special feature of the high rate of glycolysis of cancer cells is its occurrence in the presence of oxygen (aerobic glycolysis). It had been known before Warburg that many tissues, for example, muscle, can form lactic acid from glucose in the absence of oxygen (anaerobic glycolysis). All animal tissues that are metabolically active possess anaerobic glycolysis but the great majority do not glycolyse in the presence of O_2. Cancer cells differ from noncancer cells by their failure to suppress glycolysis in the presence of oxygen; a significant amount (ca. 50%) of the energy of cancer cells is derived from glycolysis under aerobic conditions. And, finally, cancer above all diseases has countless secondary causes. Almost anything can cause cancer. The prime cause of cancer is the replacement of respiration in normal body cells by a fermentation of sugar (Warburg 1969).

The findings of Warburg on metabolism of tumor cells in vitro are also valid for conditions in the intact animal. Cori and Cori 1925 studied the chemistry of blood from both axillary veins of a chicken in which Rous sarcoma had been inoculated in one wing: "If a tumor was growing on one wing, the blood that had passed through the tumor contained, as an average, 23 mg less of sugar and 16.2 mg more of lactic acid than the blood that had passed through the tissues of the normal wing."

Glycolysis was studied in liver tumors of different growth rates by Weber 1961, 1968, and 1974. Aerobic glycolysis was in the range of normal liver values in the slowly growing hepatomas; the glycolytic rate increased with the increase of growth rate and malignancy; glycolysis was high in the rapidly growing, high malignancy, poorly differentiated liver tumors.

Kubowitz and Ott 1934 were the first to isolate lactic dehydrogenase. Crystalline enzyme preparations were obtained from two sources, Jensen sarcoma of rat, and rat skeletal muscle.

From 3000 g of sarcoma (600 g dry substance) 50 mg of pure enzyme protein was obtained. From 1000 g of muscle (200 g dry weight) 200 mg of enzyme crystals was gathered. The crystals from both tissues were similar; no differences of any sort in the enzyme proteins were detected.

Goldman, Kaplan, and Hall 1964 performed electrophoresis of extracts of human and animal cancer. A definite and consistent shift was found in the pattern of molecular forms of lactic dehydrogenase (LDH) as compared with benign tumors and normal controls—there was an absolute increase in the muscle type (M4) LDH migrating negatively on electrophoresis. Meister 1950 found that the level of LDH in tumors of rodents is frequently higher than in corresponding tissues of origin.

Enzyme Patterns

The metabolic pattern is as distinguishing a feature of each living cell as is its morphology. In a classic investigation Greenstein 1947 described enzyme patterns in a wide variety of normal cells and neoplastic tissues, especially transplantable tumors, from which the following generalizations were made:

1. Each normal tissue possesses a characteristic enzyme pattern, which sets it apart from all other tissues.
2. Tumors have qualitatively the same enzymes as normal tissues.
3. Tumors possess a more uniform and less diverse chemical pattern than normal tissues.
4. When a normal tissue becomes neoplastic, many of its specific activities markedly decrease or are lost.
5. Tumors tend to converge enzymatically to a common type of tissue with nearly identical pattern. The nearly identical pattern of tumors suggests that they approach a chemically similar type of tissue.

Greenstein's law states: "No matter how, or from which tissues tumors arise, they more nearly resemble each other chemically than they do normal tissues or than normal tissues resemble each other" (Greenstein 1947).

Cell Surface Effects

Abercrombie 1961 observed that cancer cells lack "contact inhibition" in tissue culture, an effect that explains the universal propensity of infiltration of malignant growths into the normal tissues of living creatures. Normal fibroblasts seeded on a glass surface in tissue culture move predominantly out of the explant. When normal diploid fibroblasts collide, cell movement in the forward direction stops; the cells do not heap up but they form a monolayer; it is evident that an interaction has occurred and this is designated contact inhibition. In the monolayer resulting when diploid cells become confluent, the growth rate of the cells decreases markedly. In consequence an upper limit is set for the population of a given diploid cell culture which is not determined by the properties of the medium but by the inhibitory effect of cell contact.

The growth of sarcoma is quite different. When a sarcoma cell runs head on into fibroblasts, it continues its motion unimpeded, moving over or through the normal cells; the malignant cells pile up aggregating as plaques instead of forming a monolayer.

It is well established that abnormal numbers of chromosomes (heteroploidy) and progression to malignancy frequently, perhaps invariably, occur in tissue culture. Tissue culture is carcinogenic (Earle and Nettleship 1943; Sanford, Likely, and Earle 1954; Warburg, Gawehn, and Geissler (1958). Under conditions of monolayer tissue culture in unagitated flasks, the type of metabolism characteristic of malignant cells developed in normal mouse kidney cells within a few weeks (Warburg, Gawehn, and Geissler 1958).

Levine et al. 1965 found that human cell lines in which contact inhibition of growth is not operative (in general, heteroploid cells) form multilayered sheets in stationary culture and attain population densities up to ten times those of human diploid cells. Further, Levine et al. 1965 showed that in cultures of human diploid fibroblasts the rates of synthesis of DNA, RNA, and protein per cell are progressively depressed as the culture becomes confluent and that the decreases are associated with the disappearance of most of the free cytoplasmic polyribosomes. The changes are completely and rapidly reversed on subdivision of the culture.

Lectins

Certain proteins found primarily in the seeds of plants (Sharon and Lis 1972) bind specifically with sugars on cell surfaces causing the cells to clump. These aggregating proteins, designated phytohemagglutinins (PHA) or lectins, are immensely important in the study of normal and cancer cells, respectively; erythrocytes and tissue culture cells have been studied extensively.

Many important cellular functions are mediated by the surface membrane of animal cells and more particularly by branching sugar molecules, which stud the cell surface. Among the functions controlled by the surface of the cell are regulation of cell growth and differentiation, phenotypic expression, the immune response, and contact-inhibition of growth and metabolism.

The cell membrane is a bilayer of lipid molecules each with a water-soluble head and a water-repellent U-shaped double tail. Protein molecules lie on the surfaces, inner and outer, of the bilayer or are embedded in it. Some of the proteins are glycoproteins with branching chains of oligosaccharides to which particular lectins can bind. Agglutination results from cross linking of cells by lectins, which bind to specific receptors that are sugar units which protrude from the cell surface. Agglutination is inhibited or prevented if the monosaccharide that is responsible for binding to the lectin is added to a cell suspension because the monosaccharide occupies and preempts binding sites on the lectins.

Aub, Tieslau, and Lankester 1963 discovered that the supernatant of heated wheat germ lipase caused the agglutination of tumor cells, whereas normal cells did not mutually associate. The tumor cells were attracted rapidly to form a tightly bound mass which, once formed, was not disassociated by agitation or the addition of proteolytic enzymes. Lipase was not responsible since heat inactivation of the enzyme did not destroy the agglutinating activity of the preparation. Aub, Sanford, and Wang 1965 found that all leukocytes, normal and malignant, were agglutinated to some extent by wheat germ lectin. When exposed to the agglutinin, leukocytes from patients with lymphocytic leukemia consistently clumped less than those from healthy persons, whereas leukocytes from patients with granulocytic leukemia aggregated to a greater extent than those of normal controls. Agglutination is a cell surface phenomenon.

Burger and Goldberg 1967 isolated from wheat germ extracts a pure glycoprotein, which is a specific agglutinin for neoplastic cells. The tumor specific surface site which interacts with the agglutinating glycoprotein contains N-acetylglucosamine (GlcNAc). Agglutination is rapidly reversible; 10–20 seconds after adding GlcNAc the agglutinated cells begin to disperse and after 1 min previously heavy clumps disappeared to form homogeneous cell suspensions.

In the experiments of Burger and Goldberg 1967 suspensions of normal fibroblasts (BHK) did not agglutinate in the presence of GlcNAc, whereas the same cells transformed with polyoma virus did clump. Here the mother cell is differentiated only by the virus transformation from the daughter cell which possesses GlcNAc agglutination sites. Burger 1969 found that several tissue culture cell lines that had been transformed by a tumor virus reacted with an agglutinin, whereas under identical conditions their untransformed parent cell lines did not agglutinate. Remarkably, a short treatment of the parent cell line with low concentrations of proteases exposes agglutinin receptor sites indistinguishable from the transformed cells. Burger 1969 proposed that both viral and chemical transformation produced changes in the architecture of the cell membrane identical to those formed by action of the proteases. It would appear that the parent cell line has hidden agglutinin receptor sites and that the virus transformation changes the cell surface so that it is available to the agglutinin. The agglutinating ability of normal cells treated with proteases under optimal conditions is identical to that of untreated virally transformed cells.

Inbar and Sachs 1969 showed that the carbohydrate-binding protein, concanavalin A (ConA), can agglutinate leukemic cells and cells transformed by polyoma virus, chemical carcinogens, or x-irradiation. ConA did not agglutinate normal cells under the same conditions. The agglutination was reversed by competition with α-methyl-D-glucopyranoside, a carbohydrate that strongly binds to ConA, but not by GlcNAc, which does not bind to ConA. The treatment of cells with trypsin resulted in the agglutination of normal cells by ConA and a decrease of agglutinability of transformed cells.

Certain lectins stimulate mitosis. Nowell 1960 discovered that a glycoprotein in red kidney beans initiates mitosis in resting human small lymphocytes in tissue culture. In the presence of PHA, large blast cells formed and mitosis began, whereas in its absence cell division did not occur.

2

Changing the Cell's Phenotype with Epithelium, Virus, or Solid States

In animals different programs are established in various cell groups in very early stages of development; thereafter the generality of cells remain stable insofar as they are not changed into cells of other sorts. The special form and function of a cell are its phenotype.

At the moment of fertilization the spermatozoon, a haploid cell containing half the chromosomes, unites with an ovum carrying the other half; now there is present the full set of chromosomes of somatic cells. The genome is formed. The fertilized ovum, designated zygote, is the minimum connecting link between the generations; all of the cells of the organism are derived from the zygote. All somatic cells of an animal possess an identical complement of chromosomes, hence an identical genome and an equal potential to synthesize every kind of molecule to be formed by every sort of cell at each stage in its development during a life which may last more than a century. Yet, under normal conditions less than 1% of the genetic potential is expressed. The progeny of the zygote have become programmed, and this programming means that the cells have acquired distinctive enzyme patterns and therefore different cellular functions: this cell has memory while that cell can undergo muscular contraction whereas still another cell can synthesize steroid hormones. This sorting out of form and function to establish distinguishing characteristics is designated *differentiation*, that is, an individualistic phenotypic expression is firmly imprinted. Differentiation is a cardinal process in metazoan cells. The cell zealously protects the integrity of its program and forceful attempts of any sort to alter its phenotype most commonly result in the death of the cell—less often they cause cancer. Cancer is an abortive effort of a cell to change its program.

The change from a normal cell into a cancer cell can be brought about in nearly all kinds of animal tissues and by many different procedures. The change of a normal cell into a normal cell of another sort has been accomplished only in the case of a single cell type, the fibroblast (mesenchyma, stem cell of connective tissue). In this remarkable change of program by experimental means the visible and biochemical characters of the altered cells are changed so profoundly that we refer to the phenomenon as physiologic transformation; it is reminiscent of embryonic differentiation.

The physiologically transformed cells are not malignant: no tumor forms when the altered cells are transplanted into another animal; invasion and metastasis do not occur and their microscopic appearance and metabolism resemble those of normal cells. The responding fibroblasts, possessing a labile phenotype capable of alteration, are identified functionally by what they do and by their location, not by their appearance. After transformation the responding cells emerge as chondroblasts or osteoblasts; their phenotype, and that of their progeny as well, is altered permanently. The capability of responding fibroblasts in an animal to undergo physiologic transformation is present lifelong; the experimental effects are spectacular and demonstrable with regularity and ease.

Three sorts of transformation of fibroblasts will be considered: (*i*) normal fibroblast to normal osteoblast, (*ii*) normal fibroblast to malignant fibroblast, and (*iii*) normal fibroblast to malignant osteoblast.

Transforming Epithelium: Normal Fibroblast to Normal Osteoblast

The remarkable mutability of the phenotype of fibroblasts which permits a radical change of their program was discovered in the dog. In experiments on canines the surgical approximation of bladder epithelium with fascia of the trunk or limb results in the production of a large piece of bone within 3 weeks; cartilage is not observed.

In a classic experimental study Harold Neuhof 1917 investigated the possibility of repair of surgical defects in viscera with autogenous patches of fascia (connective tissue) and found that restoration indeed was possible. The closure of large defects in trachea, stomach, and other organs by sewing in a sheet of fascia was successful. The patches healed in and their fibroblasts proliferated to serve as a floor for a carpet of ingrowing epithelium. The patched organs were air- and water-tight.

An anomaly was found in the bladder, where bone regularly was found in the fascia transplant. It was significant that osteogenesis always occurred in that portion of the patch in contact with urine. Neuhof 1917 concluded that contact of fibroblasts with urine caused the formation of bone; this hypothesis was intriguing but, alas, incorrect.

In an experiment that yielded an unequivocal result, Huggins 1930 found out that bone formed in fascial patches in the empty bladder devoid of urine, which had been permanently diverted by cutaneous ureterostomy (fig. 2.1); the ingrowing epithelium had transformed the proliferating fibroblasts of the patch into osteoblasts.

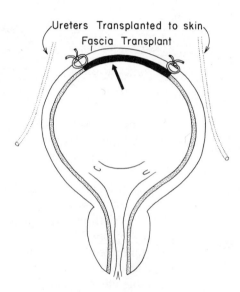

Fig. 2.1. Following bilateral cutaneous ureterostomy in the dog, fascia was transplanted to the dome of the bladder. The arrow points to site of bone formation (day 18).

In a second experiment (Huggins 1931) a segment of bladder mucosa was transplanted to the abdominal fascia, where it formed a cyst lined with epithelium. The transplanted epithelium constantly evokes a big mass of bone and the induced osteogenesis has a fixed geographic relation (fig. 2.2) to the cyst. The base of the cyst is formed by the original mucosa that was transplanted, whereas its dome is created by newly proliferating epithelium. Alkaline phosphatase was induced (Huggins 1969) in fibroblasts in contact with the epithelium of the dome but not the base of the cyst. Bone formed (fig. 2.3) exclusively in those alkaline phosphatase-containing fibroblasts adjacent to the proliferating vesical epithelium. This process of physiological transformation is designated *epithelial osteogenesis*.

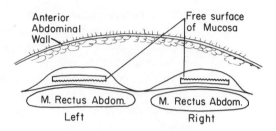

END RESULT

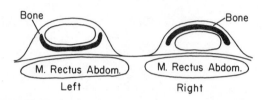

Fig. 2.2. Autologous transplantation of bladder to muscle in the dog. Above, urinary bladder has been transplanted on the left rectus muscle so that the free surface of the epithelium is toward the peritoneal cavity, whereas the mucosa of the bladder on the right faces in the opposite direction toward the skin. Below, are illustrated the epithelial-lined cysts that develop. The bone on the left is situated on the deeper aspect of the cyst, as opposed to the right, where it is on its superficial aspect. Bone always forms in the region of the newly formed epithelium.

Epithelial osteogenesis is produced invariably in fibroblasts of dog and guinea pig; in the rat, bone is evoked seldom (ca. 10% of the experiments). Three sorts of proliferating epithelium are known to be osteogenic; these are the epithelial linings of the urinary tract, the gall bladder, and the seminal vesicle (Huggins and Sammett 1933; Huggins 1969).

Bone never forms in the normal bladder of dog, despite the proximity of fibroblasts to the potentially powerful osteogenic epithelium, whereas bone always forms when vesical mucosa is transplanted to the serosal outer surface of the bladder. This remarkable effect demonstrates that, with regard to transformability, the fibroblasts are either competent or incompetent to undergo a change of program. In the urinary bladder of the dog the submucosal fibroblasts are incompetent, whereas the serosal fibroblasts on the outside of the bladder are transformed readily into osteoblasts.

Rous Sarcoma Virus-I: Transformation of Normal Fibroblasts into Malignant Ones

The origin of Rous's experiments with tumor viruses is described by the great investigator (Rous 1966):

I had done no work on cancer. I am by nature a naturalist and I was happy in my work and here I was now confronted with the unnatural which was an entirely new world to me. Suddenly there came one day a man bringing a chicken that had a lump. He had been shrugged off at two laboratories before he came to mine. They said they weren't interested and I saw my chance. He gave me the tumor and I put it through its paces.

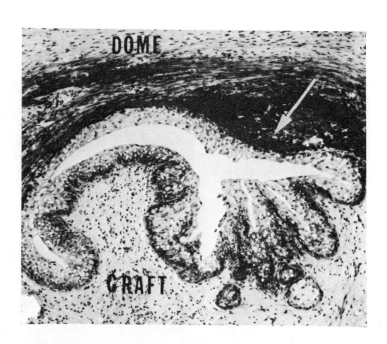

Fig. 2.3. Epithelium-lined cyst on day 12 after autologous transplantation of urinary bladder to muscle in guinea pig; the arrow points to bone that has been induced. The responsive fibroblasts in the dome are heavily infiltrated with alkaline phosphatase, whereas nonresponsive fibroblasts in the graft are devoid of this enzyme. Alkaline phosphatase stain x100.

We knew then what a tumor was like. It was a typical malignant tumor, a sarcoma. Now to transplant it, it would grow only in Plymouth Rock hens (that's a special breed); it wouldn't grow in any other that I put it into. Now this man who had brought the tumor had raised chickens because he was interested in them and had inbred them. He gave me some of his fowls and eventually let me buy for the Institute his entire stock which was closely related and I succeeded in transplanting the tumor and it grew quickly. And then simply as a duty I tried to get something out of the tumor which would cause it in other fowls. For 10 years people had been trying to get something out of transplantable tumors of mice and rats and they all failed. And to my consternation, it was very much like that, I got something out of it which would pass through a filter that would hold back bacteria. And it was a virus by all of the criteria, by all the standards, of that day. At first my critics said that I had made a mistake, that cells had slipped through the filter. I did not worry; I had the facts.

Rous 1911 was the first to isolate a virus from a solid tumor, in this case chicken sarcoma. The original sarcoma was found as a unique instance in a flock of healthy Plymouth Rock fowls. From a bit of the lump inoculated into the breast muscle of susceptible chickens there developed rapidly a large firm growth, which soon metastasized to viscera, and within 4–5 weeks the bird died. When inoculated it was at first a local disease very

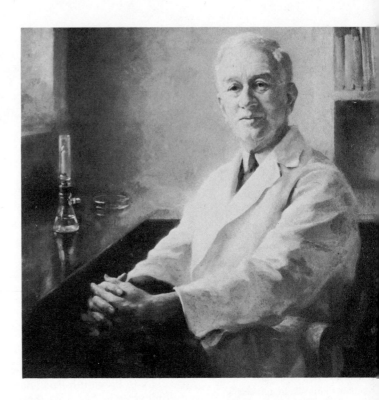

Fig. 2.4. Francis Peyton Rous
(1879–1970).

dependent on the good health of the host; at this time inter-current illness of the fowl checked the nodule's growth. Histologically the tumor always consisted of one type of cell, namely, spindle-cell fibroblasts in bundles. From the fibrosarcoma a virus, RSV-I was obtained. The secondary growths are distributed especially in the lungs, heart, and liver.

A typical experiment of Rous 1911 follows:

In this experiment the material was never allowed to cool. About 15 g of tumor from Chicken 140 (generation 7B) was ground in a warm mortar with warm sand, mixed with 200 cc of heated Ringer's solution, shaken for thirty minutes within a thermostat room, centrifugalized, and the fluid passed through a [Berkefeld] filter similar to that used in Experiment 3. Both before and after the experiment, this filter was found to hold back *B. prodigiosus*. The filtration of the fluid was done at 38.5°C and its injection immediately followed. In four of ten fowls inoculated with the filtrate only (0.2 to 0.5 cc in each breast) there has developed a sarcoma in one breast; and though the growths required several weeks for their appearance their enlargement is now fairly rapid. Pieces removed at operation have shown the characteristic tumor structure.

For almost half a century RSV-I produced only sarcomas and these in fowls. Then Zilber, Lapin, and Adgighytov 1965 reported that it would cause hemorrhagic cysts as well on inoculation into newborn rats and fibromas in rabbits. Soon it was found to give rise also to lymphomas in young rats and mice. In newborn Syrian hamsters, guinea pigs, ferrets, and monkeys it would cause fibrosarcomas (Monroe and Windle 1963).

Rous Sarcoma Virus-II: Transformation of Normal Fibroblasts into Malignant Osteoblasts

Within one year after isolation of RSV-I from a transplantable spindle-celled chicken sarcoma, Rous, Murphy, and Tytler 1912 isolated a different virus (RSV-II) from a second chicken tumor; the neoplasm was a transplantable osteochondrosarcoma.

The original tumor, an osteochondroma, appeared as a discrete mass on the sternum of an adult fowl; microscopically as well as clinically it appeared benign, but it was readily transplantable to other fowls; metastases containing cartilage were found in recipients of transplants.

A virus was isolated in the following way:

Sound portions of the tumor tissue were ground with sterile sand and taken up in a considerable bulk of Ringer's solution; shaking was done in a machine for from 20 to 30 min; centrifugalization followed and then the supernatant fluid was passed through a filter of fine texture [Berkefeld] that held back all tumor cells and was impermeable to *B. fluorescens liquefaciens*. A few cubic centimeters of the clear filtrate were injected into the trunk or leg muscles of a number of normal fowls. [Rous, Murphy, and Tytler 1912]

In the case of RSV-II, the neoplasms caused by the virus consisted, like the original tumor, of large malignant fibroblasts about which cartilage was soon laid down, followed in many instances by true bone containing red marrow.

Prior to the isolation of the osteochondrosarcoma virus, Rous had supposed that a single virus by its localization in cells of different potentiality might give rise to different sorts of tumors, but experiments with RSV-II demonstrated that the histologic character of the osteochondrosarcoma is due to a peculiarity of the causative agent which is retained when the virus is isolated from the tissue of the growth (Rous, Murphy, and Tytler 1912).

With regard to RSV-II Rous, Murphy, and Tytler 1912 wrote, "That such an agent should bring about a differentiation ordinarily foreign to the tissue is very remarkable."

Many viruses cause cancer in fowls but relatively few are known to give rise to tumors in other species, including man.

Comprehensive viruses are so called (Rous 1965) because of common attributes: each virus changes normal cells into neoplastic cells having the features which it determines, multiplies within these cells, causing what appears to be their autonomous proliferation, and can be recovered from them in a condition to produce new growths of identical sort in other similar hosts.

One might suppose that chicken tumors induced by chemical agents would also yield viral agents, but this is not so. Though they closely resemble spontaneous avian tumors in all essential particulars, a virus has almost never been procured from them (Rous 1965).

Avian Leukemia Viruses

The first tumor virus to be isolated was a myelocytic leukemia virus of chickens. This comprehensive virus, obtained from an avian myelogenous leukemia, was described in two remarkable papers by Ellermann and Bang 1908, 1909. These workers studied fowls because they were cheap, easy to procure, and were subject to leukemias that were both epidemic and endemic in this species; in addition, leukemias of this sort had never been described previously.

The chicken leukemia studied by Ellermann and Bang was characterized by an enlarged liver and spleen with involvement of bone marrow and high counts of leukocytes chiefly in the myeloid series in the peripheral blood. Microscopic investigation disclosed myelocytic involvement of capillaries in liver, spleen, and bone marrow; in liver the myeloid involvement was periportal.

In the preparations of Ellermann and Bang, pieces of liver, spleen, or bone marrow were ground in a mortar with saline to produce emulsions that were treated additionally: *i*, the organ emulsion was filtered through two layers of filter paper; *ii*, the emulsion was centrifuged and the clear supernatant passed through a Berkefeld candle filter to produce a cell-free filtrate.

The filtrates were injected in the fowls and they caused leukemias with extensive proliferation of leukocytes in capillaries, always in bone marrow, usually in liver as well. Ellermann and Bang 1908 concluded correctly, "Es muss vielmehr ein organisiertes Virus sein, dass die Krankheit hervorruft" (it must be an organized virus that calls forth the disease).

Following the injection of a cell-free filtrate, the incubation time of the leukemia was 1–2 months, but the fowls died within 8–14 days after the leukemias were recognized. Not all hens were susceptible; after a single inoculation only 40% of the recipients developed leukemia. But the immunity was not permanent; in the resistant cases multiple viral inoculations were able to evoke leukemia in those chickens in which a single dose of virus had failed to elicit the disease. One strain of virus transmitted leukemia through 6 serial passages in hens.

DNA-Containing Tumor Viruses: The Shope Papilloma Virus

Oncogenic viruses contain either double-stranded DNA or single-stranded RNA. Among the DNA-containing viruses is the papova group; the name is a mnemonic formation derived from *papi*lloma, *poly*oma, and *va*cuolating viruses. The papova group includes the Shope virus, polyoma virus, and a virus of rhesus monkey, SV40, which produces vacuoles in kidney cells. The common human wart, *verruca vulgaris*, is caused by a filterable DNA virus which is regularly and easily demonstrable in clinical patients.

In *spontaneously occurring tumors* of lower animals in which DNA or RNA viruses are implicated, infectious virus is produced by the tumors from which it is readily separable. Filterable cancer-producing agents are obtained with ease from the original spontaneous neoplasm; in fact, the virus etiology of these tumors was readily established by virtue of this property. Transplantable cancers evoked by RNA viruses retain this property, whereas the *transplantable tumors* produced by DNA viruses are usually quite different from the foregoing. Cell-free infectious DNA viruses usually are not obtained from the transplanted neoplasms. The experimental cancers produced by the DNA polyoma virus in mice failed to reveal in serially transplanted tumors the persistence of the infectious virus present in the original neoplasm (Sabin and Koch 1963).

The simian virus (SV40) causes fibrosarcomas in newborn hamsters but not in adult; the tumors can be transplanted serially and the viral genome persists but not in an infectious state (Sabin and Koch 1963). There is a close similarity between this finding and the phenomenon of bacterial lysogeny of Lwoff 1966.

Not until 1933 was a virus found that caused cancer in the mammalia. Shope 1933 discovered that a papilloma observed in wild cottontail rabbits trapped in the Great Plains of America was transmissible to both wild and domestic rabbits. The Shope virus stores well in glycerol; it is readily filterable through Berkefeld filters impermeable to *B. prodigiosus*. The Shope virus has a marked tropism for cutaneous epithelium.

The Shope papilloma is transferred with ease by rubbing the virus into scarifications made in the skin. Rabbits carrying experimentally produced papillomata are partially or completely immune to reinfection and their sera partially or completely neutralize the causative virus (Shope 1933). The disease is transmissible in series through wild rabbits. The virus of wild rabbit origin is readily transmissible to domestic rabbits, producing in this species papillomata identical in appearance with those found in wild rabbits. However, the condition is not infectious or transmissible in series through domestic rabbits (Shope 1933).

DNA-Containing Tumor Viruses: Polyoma and Marek Disease

Polyoma. Gross 1950 studied a transplantable lymphatic leukemia that originated spontaneously in a mouse of the Ak strain and was maintained by successive inoculations of leukemic cells for 52 transfers; small pieces of leukemic organs were ground in a sterile mortar and diluted with saline to obtain cell suspensions (20%) for inoculation. The age of recipients had a profound effect on transplantability. When 85 suckling mice of C3H strain, aged 1–7 days, were inoculated with Ak leukemic cell suspensions, 82 recipients developed lymphomas within 12 days. This striking susceptibility diminishes rapidly after the age of 1 week; the yield of leukemia was 0 of 58 mice inoculated at age 2–6 months (Gross 1951).

Gross 1957, 1961*a* induced leukemia in rats with a virus of high virulence (passage A) obtained from the leukemia of Ak mice. Following inoculation into newborn rats, many of the inoculated animals developed leukemias after 2–4 months.

Gross 1961*b* found that passage A virus produced not only leukemia but a diversity of tumors when it was inoculated into newborn mice. This filterable agent is now designated polyoma virus.

In the course of experiments carried out in our laboratory in 1951 dealing with cell-free transmission of mouse leukemia, filtrates prepared from spontaneous Ak leukemia were inoculated into newborn, less than 16 hours old, mice of the C3H strain. The unexpected and puzzling observation was then made that among the inoculated mice some, instead of leukemia, developed tumors on one, or both sides of the neck.

Marek Disease. Marek disease is a lymphocytic leukemia (Nazerian 1973; Purchase 1974) of chickens. It was the first neoplastic disease unequivocally shown to be caused by a herpesvirus. The most characteristic clinical signs are paralysis and emaciation. The viscera and peripheral nerves become infiltrated with leukemic lymphocytes.

Marek disease virus contains DNA and is transmissible experimentally by inoculation of visceral or blood cells of leukemic chickens. It is contagious horizontally in a flock of hens. It is stored in the feather follicles of infected fowls. It would appear that transmission is cell-associated.

Vaccination of chickens with a nonpathogenic herpesvirus of turkeys prevents leukemia even though it has little effect on the replication of Marek disease virus. The majority of the chickens that survive the infection retain lifelong the virus in their blood, leukocytes, and viscera.

RNA-Containing Tumor Viruses: Erythroleukemia and Lymphocytic Leukemia

Three filterable agents, avian sarcoma-leukemia viruses, murine sarcoma-leukemia viruses, and the mammary tumor virus (MTV) comprise the RNA-containing tumor viruses. All of them mature at the cell surface, have a high lipid content, and contain heavy RNA's (Cardiff, Blair, and DeOme 1968). The RNA's are larger than those from other groups of viruses (Benyesh-Melnick 1966). These viruses are denoted *oncorna*, derived from *onco*genic and *RNA*.

Friend Erythroleukemia. In the experiments of Charlotte Friend 1957 a cell-free filtrate of the spleen of a leukemic mouse was found consistently to cause erythroleukemia on serial passage to adult mice. Friend erythroleukemia is characterized by proliferation of immature erythroid cells which invade viscera and appear in the peripheral blood; terminally the mice have greatly elevated leukocyte counts, become anemic, and have a huge liver and spleen. The filtrates remain stable when lyophilized or stored for long periods at $-70°C$. The disease can be transmitted to adult Swiss or dba mice. Subcutaneous injection of the virus effectively reproduces erythroleukemia but tumors do not appear at the site of inoculation. The target cell is a committed erythroid stem cell.

The Friend virus, like the Gross (1961*a*) virus and other filterable agents of mouse, can transcend species barriers and produce leukemia in rat as well as in mouse. These viruses produce distinctly different diseases in mouse and rat. Mirand and Grace 1962 produced leukemias in infant Sprague-Dawley (S-D) rats by inoculation with Friend virus derived from mice: most of the recipients developed lymphatic leukemia with huge thymomas but in a few rats myeloid and erythroid leukemias were evoked.

Friend et al. 1971 found that murine virus-induced erythroleukemic cells grow well in cell suspension cultures where they exhibit a limited degree of differentiation. The cells synthesize

hemoglobin and they are malignant as tested by bioassay in
syngeneic hosts. The virus, although low in leukemogenic activity, is highly effective as an immunizing agent.

Friend et al. 1971 found that dimethylsulfoxide (DMSO)
has a striking effect on differentiation of erythroleukemia cell
lines. Of the leukemia cells permitted to grow for 4 days in a
medium containing 2% DMSO, a majority of the erythroblasts
matured to normoblasts, which stained benzidine positive. The
increase in maturation caused by DMSO or by certain highly
polar molecules or fatty acids was accompanied by an increased
synthesis of heme and hemoglobin and a decrease in the cell's
malignancy. The action of DMSO on differentiation was reversible.

Rauscher Erythroleukemia. The leukemia described by
Rauscher 1962 is characterized by a high incidence of a *dual
type* of virus-induced leukemia distinguished by rapid and extreme proliferation of erythrocytic and lymphocytic leukemic
cells, which are demonstrable as early as 7 days after inoculation. The infectious agent of Rauscher leukemia is a comprehensive virus of high virulence; RNA-virus particles of type C
are seen by electron microscopy. There is a lack of age and strain
specificity to development of Rauscher leukemias; both newborn and adult animals of many inbred and random-bred mice
and rats are susceptible. There is a short latent period before
Rauscher leukemias become manifest. Within 15 days after inoculations 50–100% of newborn or adult mice have signs of
erythroleukemia and a virulent viremia is present. Many of the
inoculated mice succumb to leukemia with tremendous enlargement of the spleen within 5 weeks. Mice surviving erythroleukemia developed lymphocytic leukemia later.

**RNA-Containing Mammary
Tumor Virus**

MTV is transferred from mouse mother to her offspring establishing a lifelong infection and virus can be recovered from
tissue or milk at any time. Little et al. 1933 discovered an extrachromosomal influence on the incidence of spontaneous mammary tumors of mice. Four big experiments were conducted
with inbred mice in which reciprocal crosses between parents of
high tumor incidence and low- or no-tumor strains were bred.
It is self-evident that in crosses of this sort the chromosomal
constitution of F_I hybrids is similar; therefore any significant
difference must be derived from outside the chromosomes.

In every instance in the experiments of Little et al. 1933, the
incidence of spontaneous mammary cancer was strikingly higher
when the cross [high tumor line ♀ × low tumor line ♂] was

made than when the cross [low tumor line ♀ × high tumor line ♂] was made in a reciprocal manner. In this way the transmission of extrachromosomal influences in murine mammary cancer was established.

In his famous foster-nursing experiment, Bittner 1936, 1942 discovered that the important extrachromosomal influence on mammary tumor development in mice was the presence of virus in milk. The experiments were conducted with newborns being nursed by foster mothers of either high or low tumor strains. In an experiment of Andervont 1940 foster nursing of C3H female mice (high breast tumor line) by C_{57} black mice (low tumor line), when the young had been with their mothers 17 hours or less, lowered the incidence of breast tumors from 100% to 25%. The first milk is not essential for breast tumor production since the virus is present in C3H milk throughout the period of lactation.

Duesberg and Blair 1966 isolated and identified the nucleic acid of MTV from the milk of nursing mice. Newly synthesized MTV-RNA was detected in mature virus particles by radioisotope incorporation [^{32}P, ^{3}H]orotic acid and identified by density gradient centrifugation and radioimmune precipitation. The MTV is a single-stranded 70S RNA. The application of these methods to monolayer cultures of MTV-infected tumor cells permitted quantitative measurement (Cardiff, Blair, and DeOme 1968) of [^{3}H]uridine incorporation into the RNA of mature MTV virus particles. In tissue culture of mammary tumor cells (McGrath 1971) replication of MTV was virtually inactive in control flasks but maturation and release of MTV by the carcinoma cells was induced by adding insulin and hydrocortisone to the culture media.

Replication of RNA-Containing Tumor Viruses

The virus of Rous Sarcoma-I is a strongly transforming C-type ribonucleic acid containing virus that replicates in vivo and in cell cultures of infected fibroblasts. How do the RNA virions reproduce themselves? In independent studies the biosynthetic mechanisms were elucidated ingeniously by Baltimore 1970 (fig. 2.5) and by Temin and Mizutani 1970.

Baltimore 1970 studied the Rauscher mouse leukemia virus setting out to look for a DNA polymerase.

With little difficulty, I was able to demonstrate that virions of Rauscher virus contained a ribonuclease-sensitive DNA polymerase activity, and, after confirming the results with Rous sarcoma virus, I knew that the machinery for making a DNA copy of the RNA genome was wrapped up inside the virions of

Production of the Integrated
Viral Genome

Expression of the Integrated
Viral Genome in a Productive Infection

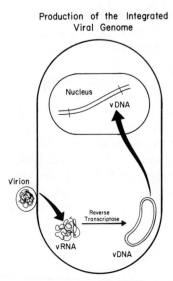
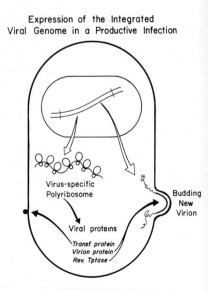

Fig. 2.5. The life cycle of an RNA tumor virus. On the basis of present knowledge, the life cycle of an RNA tumor virus can be separated into two parts. In the first part the virion attaches to the cell and somehow allows its RNA along with reverse transcriptase to get into the cell's cytoplasm. There the reverse transcriptase causes the synthesis of a DNA copy of the viral RNA. A fraction of the DNA can be recovered as closed, circular DNA and it is presumably that form which integrates into the cellular DNA. Once the proviral DNA is integrated into cellular DNA it can then be expressed by the normal process of transcription. The two types of product which have been characterized are new virion RNA and messenger RNA. Much of the messenger RNA which specifies the sequence of viral protein is of the same length as the virion RNA, but there may also be shorter messenger RNA's. The virus-specific proteins have two known functions: one is to transform cells, which occurs when, for instance, a sarcoma virus infects a fibroblast; the second is to provide the protein for new virion production. The transforming protein is shown here as acting at the cell surface, but that is only a hypothesis; *v*, viral; *Transf.*, transforming; *Rev. Tptase*, reverse transcriptase. Baltimore 1976; reprinted by permission. © 1976 by The Nobel Foundation.

RNA tumor viruses. Simultaneously with my work Temin and Mizutani discovered the DNA synthesis activity in Rous sarcoma virus. [Baltimore 1976]

Purified reverse transcriptase has the properties of most DNA polymerases: it is a primer-dependent enzyme that makes DNA in a 5' ⟶ 3' direction using deoxyribonucleoside triphosphates as substrates and taking the direction of a template for determining the base sequence of the product.

The virus-specific proteins have two known functions: one is to transform cells; the second is to provide protein for new virions.

Virus Transformation of Fibroblasts in Tissue Culture

Polyoma and simian virus 40 are small viruses that contain double-stranded DNA encapsulated in a protein envelope. These viruses induce tumors in rodents and alter the characteristics of certain fibroblasts growing in tissue culture. Homogeneous stable continuous lines of fibroblasts growing in culture have been established which are transformable in the test tube by polyoma (Macpherson and Stoker 1962) and SV40 (Todaro and Green 1963).

Stable Cell Lines. Fibroblasts are the easiest cells to grow and manipulate in cell culture and they are transformable; heritable changes can be induced in them by viruses as well as physiologic means. Fibroblasts are heterogeneous when first cultured and at this stage cannot be grown from single cells as pure clones. Experiments were performed by Macpherson and Stoker 1962 to establish stable lines of fibroblasts. A stable line is simply a mutation selected for growth in culture which can be cloned and propagated readily for many generations *and* which can be transformed in vitro by a tumor virus. Fibroblasts from baby hamster kidney were carried for several months in serial cultivation; one of the stable lines, designated BHK21, proved to be particularly useful in viral transformation studies. Fibroblasts from line BHK21 were originally cultured for 30 days, stored at $-70°$ for 60 days, and then recultured for 35 days more. The cells are fast-growing and bipolar; they grow in a monolayer with a well-marked tendency to parallel orientation; their karyotype is not abnormal. But fibroblasts in the stable line BHK21 are not completely normal since sarcoma develops when they are reintroduced subcutaneously into hamsters (Montagnier 1968; Stoker 1972). It has been pointed out earlier (p. 10) that tissue culture is carcinogenic.

Viral Transformation of BHK21 Cells. When fibroblasts from the early culture passages of stable line BHK21 were exposed to stock polyoma virus containing large quantities of virus, 33 to 73 transformed colonies were found for each 10^6 cells plated. The use of cloned hamster cell lines susceptible to polyoma transformation has provided permanence and precision in investigation because all three variables, stable cell lines, virus, and culture medium, can be preserved by freeezing.

When a fibroblast is infected with a DNA-oncogenic virus, new genetic material is introduced into the cell where it becomes integrated with the cell's DNA. The viral DNA becomes a provirus; it establishes a covalent bond (Dulbecco 1976) with cellular DNA so that each time the cell divides it copies its own DNA and the viral DNA.

Attributes of Viral-Transformed Fibroblasts. The most reliable test of true oncogenic transformation of any cell is the
ability to produce a tumor when inoculated into the proper animal recipient. Stable cell lines that have been transformed by
infection with polyoma or SV40 have special characteristics, including altered morphology, electrochemical changes in the cell
membrane, and new antigenic proteins.

1. Morphology: Untransformed fibroblasts have elongated
slender bipolar cell bodies with distinctive narrow processes; as
they multiply and crowd together, they line up in parallel bundles. Transformed cells lose their spindle-shaped bodies, become polygonal, and show random nonparallel orientation and
overlapping; they form a colony (focus).

2. Loss of contact inhibition: Normal fibroblasts show a definite migration in a monolayer. Inhibition of this movement is
found on contact of such cells with each other or with a rigid
surface. As a consequence of contact inhibition of movement the
fibroblasts orient in parallel arrays. Further, when all available
surface is covered with normal fibroblasts cell division ceases;
it is contact inhibition of growth. In virus-transformed fibroblasts, cell division does not cease at confluence and discrete
cell foci are visible in the gross in the culture plate. The focus
resembles a microtumor. Statistical considerations show that a
focus is produced by a single virus particle; the number of foci
is a measure of the transforming titer of the virus.

3. New antigens: The best evidence for the presence of an
integrated viral genome, or at least a portion of it, in DNA
virus-transformed or neoplastic cells comes from the appearance
of new antigens. Two new antigens appear in cells infected by
polyoma or SV40. One is present in the cell surface and is
called *transplantation antigen*; the other is confined to the nucleus and is designated *T antigen.*

The transplantation antigens on the cell surface can be recognized by measuring the resistance of virus-immunized animals
to challenge with neoplastic cells. Adult animals immunized
with active polyoma virus are resistant to challenge of large
doses (10^6 cells) of transformed or tumor cells, whereas non-
immune animals develop tumors when inoculated with as few
as $10–10^2$ cells (Benyesh-Melnick 1966).

Tumor (T) antigens are present in all tumors induced by
polyoma or SV40. When 3T3 cells (a continuous line of mouse
embryo fibroblasts) are infected by SV40, a large proportion of
the cell population synthesizes T antigen. During subsequent
growth, cells that are not transformed lose T antigen and only

the transformed cells of the population continue to synthesize T antigens. These observations suggest that T antigen is important for transformation.

T antigen appears in the nucleus and can be measured by immunofluorescence or complement fixation tests employing the antibodies that develop in the serum of animals bearing large primary or transplanted tumors (Eckhart 1969).

4. Growth in soft agar gels: When cell suspensions of the cloned stable line of BHK21 fibroblasts are infected with polyoma and cultured at low cell density in a glass petri dish, colonies of two distinct morphologic types develop. Most of the colonies are small monolayers of parallel fibroblasts, but 1%–5% of the cells are transformed and consist of heaps of randomly oriented cells in disarray. Macpherson and Montagnier 1964 cultured the several sorts of cells in the relatively anaerobic conditions of soft agar gels: the transformed cells grew in large spherical colonies; the generality of the untransformed cells did not form three-dimensional masses but remained as single cells in the soft gel. The nondividing cells survived for at least 10 days in the soft gels. Fibroblasts infected with RSV-I have a similar ability to form three-dimensional colonies in soft agar (Montagnier 1968).

The electric charge on the cell surface and on the fibrillar network of the gel profoundly affects colony formations. Polyanions inhibited the growth of single untransformed cells but did not influence colony formation of transformed polyoma-infected fibroblasts (Montagnier 1968). In the experiments of Sanders and Smith 1970 low concentrations of chondroitin sulfate, ovomucoid, dextran sulfate, or heparin inhibited the growth of uninfected BHK21 cells; of these polyanions heparin was the most effective inhibitor. In the presence of native collagen the colony formation of untransformed cells is enhanced four- to fivefold. Polyionic effects of this sort are limited to the normal BHK21 fibroblasts, whereas the transformed cell manifests complete resistance to the influence of electrochemical reagents so far as colony formation is concerned.

Green et al. 1966 found that collagen synthesis in the 3T3 cell line infected by SV40 differs from the uninfected parent cell line in two respects: *i*, the viral transformants produce less collagen per unit of protein synthesized than the parent line and a second differentiated function, the synthesis of hyaluronate, is also reduced; *ii*, collagen synthesis in the transformed fibroblast is less dependent on exogenously supplied ascorbate. The first result is consistent with the decrease of specialized functions in neoplastic cells, the second with an increased metabolic autonomy.

Stable cell lines of fibroblasts transformed by oncogenic viruses have membrane changes that permit lectins to bind to the cell surface and cause agglutination (p. 11).

Solid-State Carcinogenesis with Plastics: Transformation of Fibroblasts into Sarcoma

The contact of fibroblasts with many types of insoluble plastics in living animals leads to sarcomas of various sorts in rodents and induces differentiation. It would appear that this remarkable phenomenon is a physical effect in which transfer of chemical groups from plastic to fibroblast does not take place.

It was found out (Turner 1941) that the implantation of Bakelite plastic in albino rats after many months produced fibrosarcomas. The first systematic study of the carcinogenic effect of polymers was by Oppenheimer, Oppenheimer, and Stout (1952), who implanted highly purified plastic films in the abdominal wall of rodents; the plastic films included cellophane, polyethylene, and vinyl chloride, and all of the plastics induced sarcomas in rat and mouse. Within 7 days after implantation, the plastic film became enveloped in a thin membranous sac, which persisted and it was here that sarcoma developed.

Cellophane was implanted in 50 rats; 45% of the long-term survivors developed malignant tumors, which included predominantly fibrosarcomas but also liposarcomas, osteogenic sarcomas, and other neoplasms. The first tumor was observed in 263 days. The films when implanted were clear and glossy and no changes were detected in the plastics when they were removed. The fact that glass and cotton did not evoke tumors signifies some specificity of the carcinogenic effect (Oppenheimer, Oppenheimer, and Stout 1952).

The geometry of the plastic implants is a factor in tumorigenesis. Brand, Buoen, and Brand 1969 implanted vinyl chloride acetate films, 15 × 22 mm in size, in mice; sarcomas developed in 65% of males in 9–12 months. But when pieces of plastic one-third of this size (7 × 15 mm) were implanted in a control experiment, no tumors formed within the observation period of 15 months.

Many cell types will grow when attached to a rigid surface but not in suspension in liquids, a phenomenon termed "anchorage dependence." This effect was studied by Stoker et al. 1968 by incorporating solid particles of varying sizes into gels; it was found that colonies of polyoma-transformed hamster fibroblasts of the BHK21 line formed on glass fibrils 500 μm in length but not in the presence of silica fragments, which were smaller than the cells. This experiment demonstrated the requirement for growth of a rigid surface of adequate size.

A tumor of sympathetic nerve, designated mouse neuroblastoma C1300, was grown in cell culture dishes of several sorts in the experiments of Schubert et al. 1969. When cultured in a nonadherent plastic, the cells grew rapidly, remained in suspension and retained the round morphology of the in vivo tumor line. When cells grown in suspension were transferred to culture dishes chemically treated so that they could stick, long neurite processes were sent out from the cell body. The cells become electrically excitable. Culture dishes to which the cells adhered included a commercial plastic, collagen-coated dishes, and glass. In these the following sequence was observed: within 5 min the cells were attached to the walls of the culture dish; at 15 min the cells were flattened; process formation started at 2 hr and continued for several days. Electron microscopy revealed that the processes contained neurofilaments, fibers, and dense core vesicles indicative of nerve fibers. Clearly the major, if not the only, interaction initiating differentiation is that between the cell surface and the culture dish.

3 Hormones and Cancer

In its classic tradition endocrinology is concerned with some of the most bizarre displays of nature—the giants and dwarfs, the bearded ladies and beardless gentlemen, and now, vividly, with cancers.

Thoughtful man living near a natural wonder such as the Alps or a fjord, despite familiarity with the scene, often must be awestricken by its grandeur. Following hormonal intervention, the investigator sees cancer melt away in man and animals —he has observed it before a hundred times and yet he is continually astonished by the gratifying effect. Yes, the thing about cancer is to cure it.

There are fascinating facets in the relationship of hormones to cancer, but two effects stand out above all others. First, function of a normal organ can prevent cancer in a different organ at a remote site. Hygeia controls cancer. And second, function of a normal organ is necessary for the maintenance of hormone-dependent cancer; eliminate the supporting hormone and the cancer cells succumb while their host survives. Again, control of cancer is achieved through normal physiologic function.

Mitosis is prerequisite to the origin of cancer; carcinogenic agents of whatever sort are inoperative in the absence of cell division. Cancer is an impairment of mitosis.

Development of hormonal targets from infant to mature status requires growth-promoting hormones including both peptides and steroids. In their presence mitosis is extensive and growth is exuberant; in their absence mitosis is rare and atrophy prevails.

Hormones have a decisive influence on the development and course of cancers of the hormone-responsive targets, whereas tumors of nontarget cells are affected merely to a slight extent by endocrine modifications. Hormones are factors of critical importance in the cause of tumors of the endocrine-responsive tissues; cancers of this sort are diverse in kind and enormous in frequency in man and the laboratory animals. Cancers of hormone-responsive cells can be prevented by suitable alteration of the endocrine milieu. Further, modification of the tumor-host relationship by endocrine methods leads to regression and cure of many sorts of cancers of hormonal targets (p. 165). In medical clinics as well as in laboratories the regression of hormone-responsive cancers frequently is so rapid, so extensive, and so dramatic that at times it simulates witchcraft.

In women there is a high incidence of cancers of the ovary and the secondary sex organs, especially the breast and uterus. These three sorts of tumors comprise more than 40% of malignant tumors of the human female. Many of these cancers are preventable by methods presently available. In America and Europe mammary cancer has the highest rate of incidence of any malignant tumor of either sex, whereas the most common neoplasm of Japanese women is gastric cancer with mammary carcinoma far down in the list of statistics (Segi 1960; Segi and Kurihara 1972). Among patients with cancer of the breast the distribution is children 0, men <1%, and women >99%. Obviously there is a strong hormonal component in mammary cancer. Olch 1937 observed that many patients with breast cancer have a late menopause; 50% of women with cancer of the breast were menstruating at age 50. A similar delay of menopause was found in women with adenocarcinoma of corpus uteri. It is remarkable that the rate of incidence of mammary cancer has been stable (Segi 1960; Segi and Kurihara 1972) for more than two decades despite two profound changes in the mores of modern women: breast feeding has been abandoned, and highly potent growth-promoting steroids are taken regularly by large numbers of the female population for prolonged periods in large doses to prevent conception or to alleviate menopausal symptoms. Despite the consumption of hormonally active steroids each year in ton lots worldwide, there has been no epidemic of cancer or any detectable statistical increase in its incidence.

In the female, three sorts of hormones are necessary for maturation of mammary glands from infantile to adult status: somatotrophin, estrogen, and progesterone. Whereas the ovary is the most significant site of steroid synthesis in the female, its presence is not essential to induce sexual maturity or cancer formation in steroid-dependent targets. Steroid synthesis in the adrenal cortex can be sufficient in kind and amount to permit cancer to develop in the breast. The presence of pituitary hormones is necessary for the formation of mammary neoplasms;

in short, *pituitary no, mammary cancer no*. Mammary cancer is a problem in physiology of the adenohypophysis.

Cancer does not arise at the site of injection of solutions of hormones or around implanted compressed, long-lasting pellets of endocrine active materials; hormones are not "local" carcinogens. Continuous bombardment of distant and vulnerable targets by certain hormones evokes cancer in six known sites in genetically susceptible animals. In this regard hormones differ in their action from carcinogenic aromatics, which induce cancer rapidly both at the local site of injection and remotely in the prepared mammary gland and other vulnerable targets.

Six known sites of steroid carcinogenesis and the implicated hormone are:

1. Pituitary: (Cramer and Horning 1936) estrogen.
2. Leukemia: (Lacassagne 1937; Gardner, Dougherty, and Williams 1944) estrogen.
3. Mammary cancer: (Lacassagne 1932) estrogen.
4. Kidney: (Kirkman and Bacon 1950) estrogen.
5. Uterus: (Nelson 1939; Lipschütz, Vargas, and Ruz 1939) estrogen.
6. Testis: (Bonser and Robson 1940) estrogen.

Growth-promoting steroids other than estrogens have not been implicated as direct inducers of cancer.

Mammary cancer is enormously frequent in female mice but only in certain strains; the genetic constitution is a prime factor in the induction of cancer of the mouse breast. In a classic experiment, Heston and Andervont 1944 investigated the importance of the genetic and hormonal status of two stocks of mice designated, respectively, strains A and C3H; both were high mammary tumor strains and both carried the mammary tumor virus. In strain A the occurrence of mammary cancer was almost zero in virgins in contrast to an incidence of nearly 100% in breeding females. In strain C3H both virgins and breeding females have a high and equivalent incidence (100%) of cancer of the breast. Spontaneous mammary cancer has not been observed in male mice.

In a resistant strain, C57 black mice, mammary tumors were not elicited by hormonal treatments or by intensive force-breeding (Mühlbock 1956). It is obvious that the strain differences, cardinal in significance, are due to variance in the genetic constitution.

Five Estrogens

The discovery of steroids possessing physiologic activity constitutes a chapter of science that ranks with the supreme accomplishments of creative man. In 1929, Edward A. Doisy (1893–) isolated estrone in the laboratory; it was the first active steroid to be discovered and its discovery initiated a new era in biology and medicine. The active steroids promote various great physiologic effects—estrogenic, androgenic, glucocorticoid, mineralocorticoid, and progestational. They induce and they inhibit. The hormones are of crucial significance in the cause, prevention, and cure of cancer of the breast, in animals or man.

Androgens are the hormones of maleness. By definition an androgen has the following characteristics: *i*, it causes growth of the head-furnishings of the newly hatched chick; *ii*, it induces growth of cylindrical secretory epithelium in the ventral prostate of castrate or hypophysectomized male or female rats.

Estrogens are the hormones of femaleness; they induce estrus which is a form of heat not commonly measured with a thermometer. By definition, an estrogen induces squamous epithelium with keratinization in the vaginal epithelium of ovariex or hypox rat or mouse. A single steroid can induce both androgenic and estrogenic effects simultaneously in an individual animal.

Method 3.1: To Determine Estrus

Vagina of castrate rodent is washed gently with 0.1 ml of saline using a small pasteur pipette; a drop of the washing fluid is examined microscopically at magnification ×100. Estrus is present when an abundance of sharply jagged epithelial cells are present and leukocytes are absent.

Estrogenic substances are widely distributed in nature. They have been found in plants, in rocks, and in the waters of the Dead Sea. Many of the plant estrogens are phenol methyl ethers. In contrast to a number of essential oils, fennel oil and anise oil have considerable estrogenic activity, which is ascribed to the presence of anethole (Zondek and Bergmann 1938).

Three estrogens occur commonly in the animal kingdom; each was discovered in the urine of pregnancy. Organic solvents and olive oil were useful in the original preparations. In most instances the urine was extracted with chloroform or carbon tetrachloride in a glass continuous liquid extractor, often 3–4 meters in height and in many instances the apparatus reached the ceiling of the laboratory. The large apparatus permitted the extraction of as much as 30 liters of urine in 24 hr.

Estrone was isolated at Saint Louis University from the urine of pregnant women by Doisy, Veler, and Thayer 1929. The preparations of estrone were highly refined snow-white crystalline products suitable straightaway for laboratory research and clinical investigation. The excitement that the discovery of estrone created was enormous. The use of estrone in research studies became world-wide as soon as the hormone was available.

A second estrogen, estriol, was isolated from the urine of pregnant women by Doisy et al. 1930. It is of interest that in the urine of human pregnancy estriol is more abundant than estrone is, whereas it was the less plentiful estrone that was isolated first. Estriol has three oxygen functions. The hydroxyl group at position 16 (fig. 3.1) endows the estriol molecule with physiologic properties not possessed by estrone or estradiol; estriol is an impeded estrogen (p. 39).

A third estrogen, estradiol, was isolated from the urine of pregnant mares by Schwenk and Hildebrandt 1932 and it was found to have exceptionally high estrogenic potency. The key observation leading to the discovery of estradiol was fluorescence; in concentrated sulfuric acid, estradiol has orange fluorescence, whereas that of estrone is straw-colored.

Hisaw, Velardo, and Goolsby 1953 tested the three naturally occurring estrogens for their ability to promote uterine growth in rats. Adult virgin rats, aged 100 days and weighing 190–210 gm, were subjected to ovariectomy; 7 days later the ovariex rats were injected subcutaneously with the estrogens dissolved in 0.1 ml sesame oil for 3 days and killed 72 hr after the first injection. A dose response curve was established for each estrogen. The daily dose of hormone yielding maximal increase in uterine weight was: estradiol 1 μg, estrone 10 μg, and estriol more than 20 μg.

Diethylstilbestrol is a synthetic estrogen with growth-promoting activity similar to estradiol in all quantitative and qualitative respects. DES was synthesized by Charles Dodds (1899–1974), professor of biochemistry at the Middlesex Hospital, London. Dodds became impressed by the estrogenic activity of some quite simple organic compounds; among the weak estrogens were: *p*-n-propylphenol; 4,4′-dihydroxydiphenyl; 4,4′-dihydroxystilbene. It appeared that phenolic hydroxyls had high significance in estrogenicity. Dodds et al. 1939 undertook a systematic investigation to synthesize estrogen-analogs that would resemble estradiol in shape and weight and in the possession of difunctional hydroxyl groups.

The *trans* form of DES was synthesized and fulfilled the stringent requirements, whereas the *cis* form physiologically was inactive. Monohydroxydiethylstilbene had only trace activity as an estrogen, whereas diethylstilbestrol was strongly estrogenic. Injected in male rodents, DES caused marked atrophy of testis, prostate, and seminal vesicles accompanied by very marked increase in size of the adrenal glands (Dodds et al. 1939).

In addition to equivalence to estradiol in estrogenic potency, DES is prepared easily in pure form, is not costly, possesses the immense advantage of estrogenic activity when taken by mouth and it is devoid of toxicity. DES is one of the great therapeutic agents of medicine. DES was found to inhibit the activity and cause regression of human prostatic carcinoma, and its use was the beginning of chemotherapy of cancer (Huggins and Hodges 1941).

It is noteworthy that analogs of testosterone with high androgenic activity have not been synthesized.

Polymeric Estrogenic Phosphates. Polyestradiol phosphate (PEP) (Fernö et al. 1958) and related compounds (Diczfalusy et al. 1959) are long-acting, water-soluble estrogens suitable for intravenous injection. The polymeric estrogens accumulate in reticulo-endothelial cells creating a new and widely distributed endocrine storehouse from which the estrogenic compounds slowly and constantly are released. It is shown (p. 106) that these estrogens are immensely valuable in the prevention and cure of experimental cancer.

Structure-Function Relations of Estrogens and Androgens

The hypox immature female rat is in a basal endocrine state when maintained on an estrogen-free synthetic diet. In her, the uterus, vagina, and female prostate are profoundly atrophic but retain great sensitivity to growth-promoting steroids so that weakly active compounds can be assayed with ease. In certain strains of rats prostatic glands are present in high frequency in females; in these androgenic and estrogenic effects can be detected easily; androgenic activity is denoted by cylindrical epithelium in the female ventral prostate, whereas estrogenic activity is manifest in vaginal cornification.

In the experiments of Talalay, Takano, and Huggins 1952 hypophysectomy in tube-fed rats maintained on a synthetic diet inhibited the growth of intramuscular implants of the Walker tumor to ca. 46% of controls.

Using the hypox female rat maintained on our synthetic ration as an assay system, Huggins, Jensen, and Cleveland 1954 found that ketone and hydroxyl groups at position 3 and 17 (fig. 3.1) in difunctional steroids participate in the induction of growth of uterus, vagina, and prostate but that these active

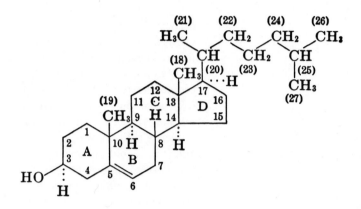

Fig. 3.1. Structural formula of cholesterol; the numbering system of steroids and sterols is presented.

centers are equivalent neither in potency nor in the pattern of growth which they evoke. The state of oxidation at both sites and the degree of saturation of the A and B rings have much to do with the quantity and type of response, androgenic or estrogenic, in the growth which steroids produce.

Butenandt and Kudszus 1935 observed that testosterone and dehydroepiandrosterone promote the growth of the comb of the capon and the prostate of male rat and also induce premature opening of the vaginal plate of immature female rats. Deanesly and Parkes 1936 discovered that dehydroepiandrosterone in addition to promoting growth of the head-furnishings of chicks induced estrus in the immature rat and caused the appearance of the female type of plumage in the Sebright bantam capon, the last effect being caused by estrone but not androsterone.

To provide a simple example of the influence of hydrogen atoms and ring-unsaturation on the pattern of hormonal activity in the hypox female rat consider 2 isomers: 4-androstene-3β, 17β-diol is an androgen that induces growth of the ventral prostate with mucification of the vaginal epithelium; 5-androstene-3β, 17β-diol is an estrogen-androgen that shares the property of the phenolic estrogens in causing keratinization of the vaginal epithelium while simultaneously inducing growth of cylindrical epithelium in the prostate (Huggins, Jensen, and Cleveland 1954).

In order to evaluate the importance of the individual structural elements of steroid hormones in accelerating growth, Huggins and Jensen 1954 investigated monofunctional steroids possessing an oxygen function at either position 3 or position 17 but not at both sites. The position of a 17β-hydroxyl group (forming androstan-17β-ol) endows the simple androstan molecule with the ability to produce growth of uterus, vagina, and prostate of the female hypox rat. It appears that hydrogen atoms at position 17 are of critical importance since related compounds with a ketone group (e.g., androstan-17-one) are inactive. Monofunctional androstan derivatives with a hydroxyl or ketone group at position 3 (e.g., androstan-3α-ol; androstan-3β-ol) are devoid of activity. If a phenolic A-ring is present in monofunctional steroids, the 17β-hydroxyl group is not necessary for growth of sex organs; proliferation of uterus and vagina followed the administration of 17-desoxyestradiol, an estrogen with a single oxygen function.

Estrogen Antagonists

The growth-promoting activity of the most potent phenolic estrogens (estrone, estradiol, DES) on the uterus can be inhibited considerably by certain antagonists. The inhibitory compounds are of two sorts: *i*, a naturally occurring hormone and closely related steroids—compounds in this class are the impeded estrogens; *ii*, synthetic compounds (fig. 3.2) which are designated anti-estrogens. These compounds have therapeutic value in the treatment of mammary cancers in some cases.

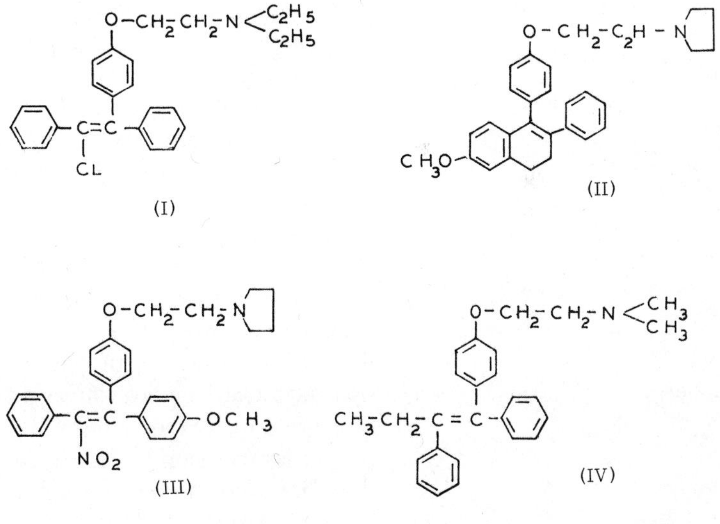

Fig. 3.2. Structural formulas of estrogen antagonists: (I) Chloramiphene; (II) Nafoxidine; (III) C1628; (IV) Tamoxiphen.

Impeded Estrogens. Possible competitive interaction of naturally occurring estrogens on uterine growth was studied by Hisaw, Velardo, and Goolsby 1953. The estrogens estradiol, estrone, and estriol were tested for effects each might have on the others vis-à-vis growth of the uterus in rats. In the combination treatments the estrogens were injected simultaneously at separate sites. The response produced by 0.1 μg estradiol or 0.8

μg estrone daily was reduced approximately 50% when combined with 1–20 μg estriol. When estradiol and estrone were given together, there was neither reduction nor summation of their growth-promoting effects; the weight increment of the uterus remained within the limits of that produced by estradiol alone. These relationships for the interaction of the three estrogens on uterine growth were in general the same when the treatments were continued for 15 days.

The observations of Hisaw, Velardo, and Goolsby 1953 were confirmed by Huggins and Jensen 1955 in hypophysectomized infant S-D rats maintained under controlled environmental conditions.

Method 3.2:
Steroid-Induced Growth
in Hypox Rat

The rats were obtained from the breeder and kept thereafter on a synthetic diet. Hypophysectomy was performed at age 24 days. The steroids were dissolved in ethyl alcohol and diluted with sesame oil. When steroids were injected in combination they were administered in the same solution, which was always freshly prepared. The solution (0.2 ml) was injected subcutaneously for 7 days beginning at age 38 days; 6–8 rats were assayed at each dose level for every compound. The perineum was observed each day for opening of the vaginal plate and cytologic smears were examined after the vagina had opened. Necropsy was performed at age 45 days at which time spleen, ventral prostate, vagina, and uterus were excised, blotted lightly, and weighed promptly on a torsion balance. Histological preparations of the vaginal epithelium were made in each case.

Impeded estrogens, members of a small class of steroids, differ from the majority of estrogenic hormones in their unusual influences on growth of the uterus. The impeded estrogens are 3-hydroxyestratriene derivatives possessing a ketone group at position 6 or a hydroxyl (α or β) at position 16. The unusual growth properties common to the impeded estrogen are twofold: *i*, after the threshold dosage required to initiate growth has been reached, the slope of the curve of increment of uterine growth in response to increased steroid dosage is very gradual rather than steep, as it is in the dose-response curve of DES, estrone, or estradiol; *ii*, the remarkable ability to inhibit to a considerable extent (fig. 3.3) the uterine growth induced by estrone administered concurrently with the impeded estrogen. The partial inhibition of estrone-induced growth of uterus is confined to a

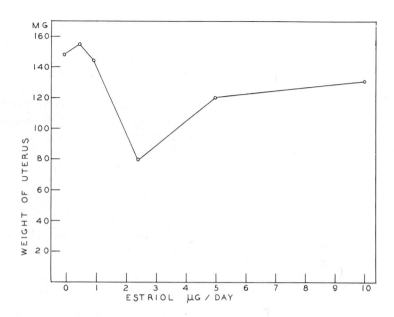

Fig. 3.3. The effect of increasing amounts of estriol administered with a constant daily amount of estrone (0.5 μg) on the weight of the uterus of hypox rats. The steroids were injected subcutaneously in the same solution daily for 7 days beginning at age 38 days. The weight of the uterus of 34 control uninjected hypox rats was 19.2 ± 2.8 mg (Huggins and Jensen 1955).

critical dosage of the impeded estrogen and is overcome by increased dosage of the inhibitory estrogenic compound. Estrone-induced growth of vagina is not inhibited by impeded estrogens. Furthermore the simultaneous administration of impeded estrogens and testosterone does not lessen the amount of uterine growth evoked by the latter.

Anti-Estrogens. Compounds in the class anti-estrogen (fig. 3.2) are related to Tace (p. xvi) in chemical structure. In ovariectomized rats the compounds are weakly estrogenic; they inhibit partially the effect of estradiol in stimulating growth of the uterus.

Holtkamp et al. 1960 administered Chloramiphene (p. xv) to young rats by daily subcutaneous injections. The compound interrupted the estrus cycle and produced metestrus; the interruption of the cycle was evident after the third injection; at this time the vaginal smear consisted of a mixture of leukocytes with only a few epithelial cells. In animals injected with Chloramiphene, the weight of the uterus was ca. 60% of that of uninjected controls and when mated with normal males they did not become pregnant.

Duncan et al. 1963 fed Nafoxidine (p. xvi) to young rats and observed the following effects: *i*, none of the animals tested in mating experiments became pregnant; *ii*, there was a slight stimulation in growth of the uterus of ovariex rats; *iii*, when administered together with estradiol, the weight of the uterus was reduced to 60% of that of rats injected with estradiol but not fed Nafoxidine.

Jensen 1965 found that Chloramiphene, Nafoxidine, and C1628 (p. xv) hindered the characteristic uptake of estradiol by target tissues in vivo. When varying doses of Nafoxidine were administered to immature rats receiving tritiated estradiol, there was a quantitative correlation between the reduction of hormone uptake by the uterus and the inhibition of its growth response. In contrast to the foregoing agents, actinomycin D and puromycin, which also block the uterotrophic action of estradiol, do not decrease the uptake and the binding of the hormone; this difference suggests that these agents act at later stages of biochemical events in which the hormone receptor interaction is the initial step.

Mechanisms of Hormone Action: Cyclic AMP

Two patterns of hormone cell interaction have been recognized (Jensen and DeSombre 1973). In the first, operative in the case of epinephrine and many sorts of peptides, the hormone reacts with nucleotide cyclase systems in the cell surface to stimulate the conversion of a nucleotide triphosphate such as adenosine triphosphate (ATP) to the corresponding cyclic monophosphate, for example cyclic adenosine 3',5'-monophosphate (cyclic AMP; see fig. 3.4). The cyclic nucleotide then serves as a "second messenger," which reacts with appropriate cellular entities to deliver and amplify the regulatory signal. Another pattern of hormone cell interaction (p. 43) is quite different from the foregoing. This pattern deals with steroids rather than with peptides or amino acids. In this mechanism, interaction with steroid receptor proteins is the primary biochemical event in hormonal action.

In a series of ingenious experiments, Sutherland 1972 discovered the significance of cyclic AMP in hormone action. The researches of the Sutherland school began with the study of the breakdown of glycogen in liver tissue brought about by epinephrine or glucagon. The glycogenolytic action of these hormones was attractive for several reasons: *i*, the effects were rapid, large, and reproducible; *ii*, liver slices could be utilized for in vitro experiments. Significantly, Sutherland 1972 found that all response to hormones was lost when the liver cells were disrupted.

Epinephrine acts on the hepatic cell to stimulate the action of adenyl cyclase, an enzyme bound to cell membranes. This augmentation leads to increased levels of cyclic AMP, which

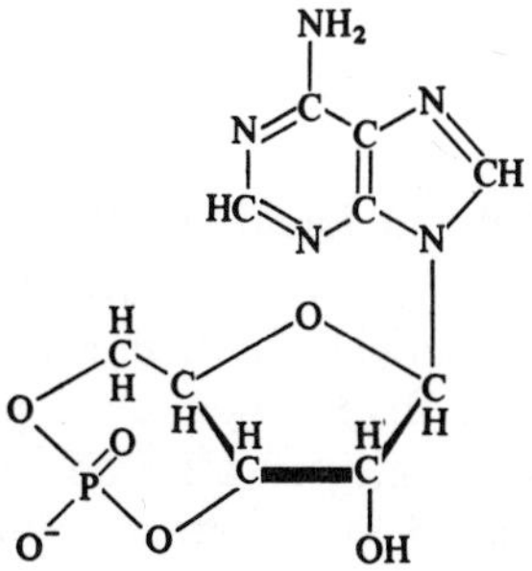

Fig. 3.4. Structural formula of adenosine 3′,5′-monophosphate (cyclic AMP).

acts intracellularly to alter the rate of one or more cellular activities. Increased cell permeability takes place. Since cells contain different enzymes in their phenotype, the end result of the hormonal augmentation of cyclic AMP differs widely from one cell type to another; for example, through the action of cyclic AMP, epinephrine causes the breakdown of glycogen in liver cells, whereas ACTH induces the synthesis of corticosteroids in the adrenal cortex. Since many hormones produce at least some of their effects by way of cyclic AMP, the involvement of this nucleotide in endocrine action is far-reaching. Of the polypeptide hormones, ACTH, LH, gonadotrophins, thyrotrophin, parathyroid hormone, and glucagon produce at least some of their effects by way of cyclic AMP.

Mechanisms of Hormone Action: Estrogen Receptors

A pattern of hormone cell interaction, operative with various types of steroid hormones, is fundamentally different from the pattern of biochemical action set in motion by epinephrine and the peptide hormones via cyclic AMP (p. 42). In the steroid pattern of interaction, the hormone enters the cell where it binds to a specific extranuclear receptor-protein characteristic of the responsive target cell. The resulting steroid-protein complex then migrates to the nucleus where specific RNA synthesis is initiated or accelerated leading in the case of the estrogenic hormones to tissue growth. The hormone-induced translocation to the nucleus involves an alteration of the receptor-protein.

A major advance in the understanding of the interaction of steroid hormones with target cells came in studies of the interaction of tritium-labeled estrogens with hormone-dependent tissues through the work of E. V. Jensen. The striking affinity for estradiol both in vivo and in vitro demonstrated that such target tissues as uterus, vagina, and anterior pituitary possess unique binding components designated estrogen receptors. Strong, but reversible, association of the hormone with receptor proteins without chemical transformation of the steroid molecule is the primary step in the uterotrophic process, not affected by such inhibitors of early estrogen response as puromycin or actinomycin D.

Jensen and Jacobson 1960 were the first to synthesize estradiol labeled with carrier-free tritium. The radioactive hormone possessed sufficiently high specific activity to allow study in the rat of the distribution of a physiologic amount of estradiol, which was injected after administration of minute amounts of [^{3}H]estradiol to immature animals; the uterus, vagina, and anterior pituitary take up and retain radioactive hormone against a large concentration gradient in the blood (Jensen and Jacobson 1962). Despite extensive metabolism of estradiol in the animal giving rise to a variety of metabolites, only unchanged estradiol is bound by uterus of the immature rat. The discovery by E. V. Jensen 1965 that estradiol binds to receptor substances and initiates growth of the uterus without undergoing chemical conversion has proved consistent with much subsequent research and served to direct investigative attention away from earlier considerations that had linked estrogen action to steroid metabolism.

Two estrogen-binding proteins possessing in common the attribute of specific and high attraction for estradiol, but not estrone, have been found in hormone-dependent target tissues. Centrifugal fractionation studies demonstrate two sites of estrogen binding in uterine cells. As confirmed by autoradiography, most of the estradiol both in endometrium and in myometrium resides in the nucleus but a certain amount is bound to a macromolecular substance appearing in the supernatant cytosol (Jensen et al. 1968).

Toft and Gorski 1966 observed that the estradiol-receptor complex in the cytosol can be characterized by ultracentrifugation in sucrose density gradients where it migrates as a discrete macromolecular band with a sedimentation coefficient at first reported as 9.5S but now known to be closer to 8S; disruption of the complex by proteases but not by nucleases indicates that the receptor substance is a protein.

Jensen et al. 1968 found that the major part of radioactivity bound to nuclei can be solubilized by salt extracts yielding a different macromolecular complex sedimenting at about 5S. The 8S complex transfers estradiol to the nucleus by a process that consumes the 8S receptor. When the 8S complex of the cytosol is exposed to the same concentration of salt solutions used to extract the nuclear complex, the 8S component is dissociated reversibly into a subunit sedimenting at about 4S and clearly distinguishable from the nuclear 5S complex by careful gradient centrifugation.

The foregoing observations demonstrate a two-step interaction mechanism (Jensen et al. 1968) in which the 4S binding subunit of the 8S protein, which is present in excess in the extra-nuclear fraction of uterine cells, serves as the uptake receptor combining directly with estradiol. This association of the hormone with receptor permits the protein to enter the nucleus by a temperature-dependent process accompanied by transformation of the 4S binding subunit of the uptake receptor to a 5S form that becomes bound in the nuclear chromatin (Jensen et al. 1971). The increase in the sedimentation rate of the complex from 4S to 5S, designated receptor transformation, includes the ability to bind to uterine nuclei (Jensen et al. 1972) and to stimulate the activity of Mg^{++} dependent nuclear RNA polymerase (Mohla, DeSombre, and Jensen 1972).

Jungblut et al. 1976 summarize the series of events in a target cell in the presence of estradiol:

i. Attachment of the steroid to the receptor, which undergoes a major conformational change when enveloping the steroid.

ii. Dimerization to steroid-receptor: receptor-steroid.

iii. Translocation of the dimer into the nucleus.

iv. Enhancement of transcription.

Hormone-Induced Growth of Mammary Gland

In the hypox rat, steroids alone are sufficient to cause growth of uterus, vagina, and female prostate, but the mammary glands are quite different from these structures. In hypox rat both peptide hormones and steroids are required for growth of the mammary tubules.

Reece, Turner, and Hill 1936 found that estrogens or testosterone failed to induce growth of the mammary glands of the hypox rat. Reece and Leonard 1941 observed that simultaneous injection of steroids and pituitary growth hormone elicited extensive lobule-alveolar growth of mammary glands of hypox rats; therefore some pituitary "mammogen" is essential for growth of rat's mammary glands. Gardner and White 1941 found the mammary gland rudiments grew in hypox male mice receiving both prolactin and estrogens. The administration of prolactin alone did not result in mammary growth.

Hyperplastic Alveolar Nodules

Alveolar nodules (HAN) are found frequently in the mammary glands of female mice of strains with a high incidence of mammary cancer. The nodules are accessible and have been studied extensively. It is generally accepted that mammary cancer of the mouse arises in the hyperplastic alveolar nodules. It is known that many of the nodules are precancerous, whereas others are established lilliputian malignant tumors, adenocarcinoma in type. In their early stages HAN are hormone dependent. In their late stages, mammary cancers of the mouse are not dependent on hormones.

DeOme et al. 1959 transplanted either HAN or samples of normal mammary tissue into mammary gland-free fat pads of isologous recipients. It was found that the hyperplastic nodules gave rise to mammary cancer more frequently and in shorter time than did normal mammary tissue.

Mühlbock 1956 studied whole mounts of mammary glands of females of the high mammary cancer dba strain of mice. Many nodules were found regularly before age 1 year in females infected with mammary tumor virus (MTV). In dba females without MTV, fewer mice developed nodules and the minimum age for their occurrence was 15 months. The incidence of nodules increased as follows: virgins < breeders < force breeders; in all dba females with MTV the occurrence of nodules was considerably higher than in virus-free mice. Mühlbock 1956 concluded that mammary cancer can develop in mice in the absence of MTV and that the mammary tumor virus is not a primary causative factor; MTV is an important accelerator of development of mammary cancer.

The influence of hormones on the development of tumors of the mammary gland of mouse has been studied comprehensively by Bern, DeOme, and Nandi at the University of California; C3H mice, which were used in the majority of the studies, bear MTV and have an incidence of mammary cancer that approaches 100% in virgin and breeding females.

Bern 1960 found that HAN do not develop in the mammary glands of hypox mice inasmuch as a tumor cannot arise in a nonexistent organ. The hormones required for normal mammary development must play an essential role in eventual tumorigenesis. In the absence of the hypophysis, estrogen alone is insufficient as hormonal replacement to permit normal development or tumor formation. Estrogen plus a pituitary peptide plus a second steroid (luteoid or corticoid) are the minimal factors to permit cancer of the breast to develop. In a genetically tumor-susceptible, virus-infected mouse, this limited degree of hormone-induced development will result in precancerous lesions in the mammary glands.

Bern and Nandi 1961 studied ductal development and the occurrence of adenomatous nodules in mice subjected to triple operations (hypox, adrenalectomy, and ovariex). The effective hormonal conditions for adenomatous nodule formation in endocrinectomized mice were the same as for lobule-alveolar development in intact animals. The administration of estrogen *plus* a second steroid (progesterone or glucocorticoid) *plus* a pituitary peptide (lactogenic hormone or somatotrophin) causes the emergence of nodules along with the development of normal alveolar lobules. Estrogen and progesterone and growth hormone are required for maximal development of lobular-alveolar growth and mammary tumors in mice.

Endocrine Induction of Experimental Cancer

Mammary Cancer in Mouse. Mammary cancer was the first neoplasm to be elicited by endocrine means (Lacassagne 1932). In mice of the Paris RIII strain, the incidence of breast cancer approached 100% in females, whereas it had never been observed in males. In the famous experiment of Lacassagne 1932, 3 male mice of this strain were injected subcutaneously once each week with estrone benzoate, 30 μg, starting at age 10–18 days; each of these males developed mammary cancer within 5 months. Lacassagne pointed out two possible interpretations: that estrone stimulation in maintaining the mammary glands permitted a latent predisposition to cancer to exert itself, or that estrone induced the mammary cancer.

Haagensen and Randall 1942 found that estrone increased the incidence of mammary cancer in male mice of a high cancer strain without increasing it in females. In this work it appeared that hormonal factors in addition to estrogen are of considerable significance in the development of cancer of the mouse mammary glands.

Since the original research of Lacassagne 1932, numerous experiments have been conducted on the influence of estrogens in the development of mammary cancer in mice. The results have been reviewed by Mühlbock 1956. It may be stated in general that the administration of estrogenic hormones is followed by the occurrence of mammary cancer in gonadectomized mice of high cancer strains when the mammary tumor virus is present; male mice are more susceptible to estrone-induced mammary cancer than females are.

Mammary Cancer in Rat. Mammary cancers sometimes occur in rats given exogenous estrogens for many months, but the incidence of the neoplasms is not high and there is a prolonged latent period before the tumors become manifest. In addition, there is a formidable disadvantage in this species which concerns big doses of estrogens. In the rat, the administration of large amounts of estrogen leads to extreme enlargement of the uterus with massive and often fatal endometritis. Prophylactic hysterectomy is necessary before estrogen treatment in order to prevent this complication.

Noble and Collip 1941 implanted pellets of estrone in newborn male and female rats; mammary carcinoma was detected in 28 of 49 rats in 226–335 days. In 4 rats removal of the pellet was followed by rapid regression of all mammary tumors (Noble and Cutts 1959). Nelson 1944 injected rats with DES, 50 μg, daily; mammary tumors were observed in 29 of 54 rats, which survived 300+ days; the first tumor was observed on day 250. Maisin, Meerseman, and Maldague 1956 implanted pellets of DES in rats that were observed for 300+ days, but no mammary cancers were found.

Huggins and Grand 1966 subjected 15 female S-D rats to hysterectomy-ovariectomy at age 40 days; beginning at age 66 days every rat was injected with 50 μg of estradiol daily for 400 consecutive days. We found that 1 rat developed mammary cancer, which was detected on day 358, whereas 14 rats remained free from cancer of the breast. Dunning, Curtis, and Segaloff 1947 demonstrated a significant strain difference in response to the implantation of estrogens in pellet form; mammary cancers developed in 3 of 4 strains, whereas one stock remained free from cancer of the breast.

Pituitary Tumors. Two ways to induce pituitary tumors experimentally are: (*i*) the long-continued administration of large doses of estrogen, and (*ii*) heavy doses of radiactive iodine.

Estrogen. Pituitary tumors were first evoked experimentally in a strain of mice with a high incidence of spontaneous mammary cancer in females, whereas none of the males developed cancer of the breast. Cramer and Horning 1936 painted the skin of male and female mice of the Paris RIII strain with a solution of estrone; all of the males but none of the females developed cancer of the breast, which arose after 16 to 21 weeks. Chromophobe adenomas were found in the pituitaries of many of the mice, both males and females, after prolonged treatment with estrone.

Gardner 1948 studied the induction of tumors of the anterior hypophysis in strains of mice which were injected with large doses of estrogens. Pituitary tumors developed in highest incidence in the C57 black mice, a strain with low incidence of spontaneous mammary cancer. Estrogenic treatment of mice of six other strains rarely elicited pituitary tumors. Chromophobe adenomas arose in localized areas of hyperplasia in the pituitaries; at times the tumors attained the size of a normal mouse brain. The tendency for estrogen treatment of C57 black mice to induce pituitary adenomas is transmitted genetically by both males and females to their hybrid offspring. Simultaneous administration of androgen with estrogen reduced the incidence of pituitary adenomas.

In albino rats, pituitary adenomas arise after prolonged treatment with large doses of estrogens; the pituitary tumors produce exophthalmos when they attain large size and the size of the head increases.

Radioactive Iodine. Gorbman 1950 injected mice with doses of ^{131}I, sufficient to destroy the thyroid gland and thereby to curtail body growth. About 8 months after the thyroid-lethal doses of ^{131}I more than 90% of the mice had developed neoplasms of the pituitary; the tumors were noninvasive. Mice of the C57 black strain had long periods of vaginal cornification and presented other evidence of high levels of circulating estrogens.

Furth and Burnett 1951 observed that pituitary tumors induced by thyroid-destructive doses of ^{131}I are readily transplanted into mice whose thyroid glands have been destroyed but not in normal mice. The pituitary growths are conditioned tumors formed by cells driven to proliferation by the lack of thyroid feedback hormones. The mice with pituitary tumors had conspicuous enlargement of ovaries and uterus; the same chromophobe cell in mouse pituitary can synthesize both gonadotrophic and thyrotrophic hormones.

Adrenal Tumors in Mouse. C. C. Little (1888–1971), American geneticist, was tall, handsome, boundless in energy, and highly intelligent; he possessed great personal magnetism and leadership and so a school formed around him. As an experimentalist Little was innovative and persistent in the pursuit of interesting new knowledge. His many contributions to science were characterized by simplicity and elegance.

Little and his co-workers found that there is an easy way to produce tumors of the adrenal cortex. The method involved selection of a suitable strain of mice and removal of the gonads soon after birth. In such animals there developed adrenal hyperplasia followed by benign and malignant tumors of the adrenal cortex. The excessive activity of the adrenal stimulated the development of uterus and mammary glands in older animals so that mammary carcinoma formed in many of the gonadectomized mice.

Woolley, Fekete, and Little 1939 removed the ovaries of a dilute brown strain of mice, designated JAX-dba, soon after birth. At 6 months in these animals the uterus was thin and threadlike but several months later it underwent hypertrophy; some mice developed estrus cycles. At 6 months the mammary tubules showed no growth; beyond one year there was extensive duct development accompanied by mammary adenocarcinoma. The incidence of mammary cancer in JAX-dba mice was: virgin females 50%, one ovary removed 39%, and bilateral ovariectomy 27%. The adrenals in castrate females were enlarged and contained yellow nodules. In brief, the prolonged action of the hyperplastic adrenal resulted in maturation of the mammary glands and uterus and the development of cancer of the breast. Adrenal function simulated ovarian activity.

In ovariectomized females the histology of the submaxillary glands was masculine in type (Woolley and Little 1945b) in contradistinction to the characteristic feminine histologic appearance in intact female controls. Few anatomic abnormalities were found in the pituitary glands. Ferguson and Visscher 1953 found that hypophysectomy prevented the development of postcastrational hyperplasias and adenomas in the adrenal cortex in male and female mice.

Woolley and Little 1945a found that gonadectomy led to adrenal tumors in male mice as it did in females and to mammary cancer in both sexes. The development of adrenal cortical hyperplasia and tumors was not uniform in all mice strains. There was considerable development of adrenal hyperfunction with maturation of secondary sex organs in gonadectomized mouse strains characterized by a high incidence of spontaneous mammary cancer, including the strains dba and C3H. There was a low incidence of both adrenal tumors and spontaneous mammary cancer in the C57 black strain of mice.

In a strain of mice designated JAX-ce, Woolley and Little 1945a, b found that neonatal gonadectomy led to malignant tumors of the adrenal cortex. In this strain the incidence of adrenal cortical carcinoma at age 6 to 12 months was: intact control females, 0 and ovariex, 100%; intact control males, 0 and castrate males, 79%.

The formation of adrenal cancer following removal of the gonads in early life is a regulated function. *The presence from birth of ovary or testis prevents adrenal cortical carcinoma.*

Woolley and Little 1946 observed that adrenal cortical adenomas and carcinomas of mice that had been gonadectomized soon after birth did not appear in mice treated with stilbestrol. Fusion pellets of DES in cholesterol, average weight 4.8 mg were implanted subcutaneously on a single occasion when the mice were age 7 weeks. The stilbestrol-treated mice of both sexes observed up to 14 months did not develop adrenal tumors.

Leukemia in Mouse. Lacassagne 1937 observed that many mice of the Paris RIII stock developed leukemia when subjected to prolonged treatment with estrogens. Gardner, Dougherty, and Williams 1944 subjected mice of 7 strains to injections of estrogens for prolonged periods ranging from 10 weeks to many months. The incidence of tumors among untreated control mice of the different strains ranged from 0 to 5%; of 1799 companion mice treated with estrogens, 215 (11.9%) acquired leukemia. The combined administration of testosterone with estrogens reduced the frequency of leukemia to that of untreated controls.

Endocrine Prevention of Cancer

Moore and Price 1932 discovered that the injection of estrogen abolished castrational changes in rat's pituitary and diminished gonadotrophin production. This important observation established a principle of endocrinology: There is a reciprocal regulatory relationship between endocranial and exocranial hormones whereby the products of endocrine glands regulate the production of pituitary trophic hormones and vice versa. This relationship is analogous to a closed cycle feedback circuit much used in servomechanisms.

There are three endocrine methods to prevent cancer of hormonal targets:

i, elimination of excessive hormonal stimulation—this was achieved by Lathrop and Loeb 1916 by ovariectomy;

ii, furnishing hormonal feedback; and

iii, competitive inhibition with hormones.

Mammary Carcinoma. Ovariectomy in adolescent mice leads to a considerable decrease in the incidence of mammary cancer and a delay in the appearance of the tumors. Lathrop and Loeb 1916 stated, "If mice are castrated at or below the age of 6 months the tumor incidence will be markedly diminished; we found it decreased from between 60 and 70% in the controls to 9% in the castrated mice."

Cori 1927 investigated the influence of ovariectomy performed at age 15–22 days on 100 mice of the Marsh Buffalo (high mammary cancer) strain. At age 20 months the incidence of spontaneous mammary cancer was: control virgin females 74% and ovariex, 0.

Ovarian Tumors. Biskind and Biskind 1944 observed that autologous transplantation of an ovary to the spleen with contralateral ovariectomy led to the development of ovarian tumors in rats. A regular sequence of events occurs after intrasplenic ovarian transplants in castrate rats: in the ovary there is a constant development of new follicles that luteinize; subsequently granulosa cell tumors and luteomas form. In these rats the pituitary is of the castrate type and the uterus is atrophic. The portal circulation from the spleen leads the ovarian estrogens to the liver, where they are inactivated; since the feedback steroids from the ovary are destroyed, the pituitary misreads the hormonal status of the organism, interpreting it to be deficient in steroids and so increases gonadotrophin production. The development of tumors in an intrasplenic ovary was prevented by administration of estrogen or by retention of the contralateral normal ovary in its usual site in the abdomen (Biskind, Kordan, and Biskind 1950). *The presence of one normally functioning ovary prevented cancer in both ovaries.*

Endocrine-Induced Remission of Cancer

The cure of cancer by alteration of the endocrine milieu is without danger, and it is not toxic. Remarkably, the benefits can be evident within a few hours, and they can persist lifelong. There can be complete and permanent disappearance of the lesions.

The control of cancer by endocrine methods has been described (see appendix 1) in three propositions (Huggins 1967), which constitute a paradigm:

1. Some types of cancer cells differ in a cardinal way from their nonmalignant ancestors in their response to changes in their hormonal environment.

2. Certain cancer cells are hormone-dependent and these malignant cells succumb when deprived of supporting hormones.

3. Certain cancer cells succumb when excess amounts of hormones and related compounds are administered.

In hormone-responsive cancers appropriate endocrinologic modification results in catastrophic effects on malignant cells of several kinds in man and the animals, even in those in the terminal stages of the disease.

Mammary Cancer and Oophorectomy. The first indication that advanced cancer of any sort could be induced to regress by any method was the beneficial effect of removal of the ovaries on two women with cancer of the breast. The observation of Beatson 1896 was remarkable since it was made before any concept of endocrine secretions had been developed.

Prior to his great discovery at the Glasgow Cancer Hospital, Beatson 1896 studied lactation in farm animals.

It is just twenty years ago that I was asked to take medical charge of a man whose mind was affected, and I went to reside with him at one of his estates in the west of Scotland.

My duties were at times exciting, but never onerous and I had a good deal of leisure to myself. I thought it would be a good opportunity of writing my M.D. thesis, and after consideration I decided I would take up the subject of lactation.

The first patient subjected to ovariectomy was a woman, age 33, suffering from a large recurrent fungating cancer of the breast. Improvement after removal of the ovaries was rapid, dramatic, and long-lasting (Beatson 1896).

Eight months after my operation all vestiges of her previous cancerous disease had disappeared. The conclusion I draw from the two cases I have brought under notice is this—that we must look in the female to the ovaries as the seat of the exciting cause of carcinoma, certainly of the mamma, in all probability of the female generative organs generally.

Mammary Cancer and Bilateral Adrenalectomy. It was found out (Huggins and Bergenstal 1951, 1952) that removal of the adrenal glands with maintenance of the patient by means of glucocorticoids can cause regression of far advanced mammary cancer in clinical patients. There were three theoretical considerations leading to adrenalectomy: *i*, gonadectomy in mice is followed by a compensatory hypertrophy of the adrenal, increased cortical function, and mammary cancer (Woolley, Fekete, and Little 1939); *ii*, in men orchiectomy is followed by increase in 17-ketosteroids and the high values are eliminated by adrenalectomy; and *iii*, following oophorectomy women continue to excrete estrogens in the urine. *The adrenals are the gonads of the aged*.

Huggins and Dao 1952 devised a simple and safe surgical technique for total adrenalectomy in the human in one seance. An essential factor in adrenal surgery is the prevention of adrenal insufficiency during and after the surgical operation. Huggins and Bergenstal 1951 formulated a medical regime by which Addison's disease of surgical origin is regularly prevented. It was found out that total adrenalectomy benefited patients with Cushing's disease and those with mammary cancer.

Concerning adrenalectomy as a treatment for human breast cancer, Cade 1955 stated, "In a proportion of cases both subjective and objective improvement has been achieved which has never been accomplished before by any other method of treatment."

Mammary Cancer and Hypophysectomy. Luft and Olivecrona 1953 performed hypophysectomy in 12 cases of malignant tumors; the operation was well tolerated in every case, and there were no deaths or serious complications. Objective improvement was seen in two patients, one with malignant chorionepithelioma, the other with mammary carcinoma.

Pearson et al. 1956 carried out surgical ablation of the hypophysis in 79 cases with advanced cancer by way of a frontal craniotomy. Objective evidence of remission was obtained in 21 out of 41 cases of mammary cancer. In this group of patients Pearson et al. 1956 observed regression of primary inoperable lesions and of metastases in many locations.

Mammary Cancer and Estrogens. A half century after the classic observation of the beneficial effect of ovariectomy (Beatson 1896) on mammary cancer, Haddow et al. 1944 found that estrogens can have an ameliorative action in human mammary cancer. A paradox seemed to be involved since, in some circumstances, estrogens were apparently activating agents for cancer of the breast. In one room the surgeons were removing sources of estrogenic hormones, while nearby the physicians were prescribing estrogens for mammary cancer. The vexatious paradox was solved by experimental studies.

The following changes occur in patients with advanced cancer of the breast treated with estrogens (Nathanson 1947): ulceration of the primary cancers can decrease in size or heal; masses regress significantly; skin nodules and lymph nodes become smaller; and regression of pulmonary or osseous lesions may occur. Side effects from estrogenic treatment (Huggins 1954) are edema, vaginal bleeding, nausea and vomiting, pigmentation, hypercalcemia, and incontinence.

Obligatory Growth

The hormone-supported growth of target cells is mandatory even in highly disadvantageous physiologic states such as prolonged and complete absence of dietary nitrogen. Pazos and Huggins 1945 found that the prostate grew exuberantly in immature castrate dogs deprived of all food, given water to drink, and injected with testosterone; the increase in mass of the prostate was fourfold after 21 days of starvation, during which the dogs lost 40% of their body weight. Testosterone confers on the secondary sex organs of the male a nutritional advantage whereby these organs grow utilizing as substrates the products of the calamitous general tissue breakdown of prolonged inanition.

Mammary Cancer in Dog and Adrenal Cortical Tumors

Mammary carcinoma is a frequent disease of elderly female dogs but it is rare in male canines. The mammary tumors of dogs are multiple; in a series of 31 dogs with cancer of the breast, 120 mammary growths of appreciable size were counted.

The neoplasms frequently metastasize. The dog with mammary tumor has many endocrine abnormalities (Huggins and Moulder 1944).

There are three distinctive attributes of mammary cancer in the canine species: *i*, there is a significant association with tumors of the adrenal cortex; *ii*, most of the mammary cancers secrete milk persistently; and *iii*, bone is found in many of the mammary cancers.

Female dogs have a characteristic functional reproductive sequence; pseudopregnancy occurs in virgin dogs twice each year. Vaginal bleeding and lactation occur at regular intervals; ovulation is spontaneous; corpora lutea form in the ovary and the luteal phase is long in duration. Most of the mammary cancers lactate persistently (Huggins and Moulder 1944).

In a series of 31 dogs with cancer of the breast, every animal was found to have bilateral adrenal tumors. The neoplasms encroach upon the adrenal medulla and fungate through the surface of the adrenal cortex; many of the tumors are of considerable size and their cells contain much lipid. Lactation continues in the majority of dogs despite removal of both the ovaries and the adrenal glands.

Bone and cartilage, occurring as minute spicules or large dense masses, were found in the mammary cancers in 8 of 31 dogs. It was found out that bone in the tumors arises through the process of epithelial osteogenesis (Huggins and Moulder 1944).

4

The Road to 7,12-DMBA and 7,8,12-TMBA

Although any intervention that can alter the genetic code without destroying it will cause cancer under fitting conditions, certain chemical compounds are more effective than others in this regard; these are termed carcinogens. Some of the chemical carcinogens are extremely powerful and rapid in their action; the most active compounds are polycyclic aromatic hydrocarbons and aromatic amines. It is thought that many of these carcinogenic substances act directly on the cell without chemical change, whereas others may require preliminary metabolic activation to render them capable of causing cancer. In their ability to evoke cancer in rodents, 7,12-DMBA and 7,8,12-TMBA and a few of their congeners exceed by a factor of 2 or more all other hydrocarbons (Bachmann, Kennaway, and Kennaway 1938). In addition, 7,12-DMBA and closely related compounds inflict unique kinds of lesions in the adrenal cortex and testis (p. 130) which set them apart from other chemical substances.

In a useful paper Bachmann and Chemerda 1938 described the synthesis of 7,12-DMBA and 7,8,12-TMBA, the most powerful of the chemical carcinogens. These compounds are reagents that act on cells during synthesis of DNA (Ford and Huggins 1963; Jensen, Ford, and Huggins 1963). Both compounds evoke cancer when applied to the skin, fed by mouth, inserted in the colon (Huggins, Morii, and Grand 1961), or injected into susceptible mice or rats, purebred of every strain or random bred, of both sexes, and of all ages; good health is required in the recipient for carcinogenesis. Any change in the structure of these compounds leaves unaltered the carcinogenic potency of 7,12-DMBA and 7,8,12-TMBA or results in a decrease of it; no metabolic change is known to enhance the cancer-producing activity of the parent compound.

The syntheses of the outstandingly powerful carcinogens represent the successful completion of a hot chase by talented chemists working in cooperation with biologists, surgeons, and pathologists. Science is people: as the work progressed, there were profound mood changes in the investigators, running the gamut from exhilaration to depression as new facts confirmed, modified, or destroyed a hypothesis. It was a detective story carried out in four countries over 162 years. The story is as entrancing as one of the tales of Scheherazade.

Human Cancer Caused by Soot

The writings of Percivall Pott, a famous London surgeon, on many subjects have had a profound effect on clinical surgery. His paper, "Cancer Scroti," (Pott 1808) was the beginning of modern cancer research, appearing as a sudden sunrise dispels an inky night.

Percivall Pott (1713–88) was apprenticed in 1729 to a barber-surgeon at Saint Bartholomew's Hospital, where he served with distinction for almost six decades. He often arrived at the hospital dressed in a red coat and wearing a sword (Morgan 1968). Among his pupils was John Hunter; his patients included Dr. Samuel Johnson and David Garrick.

Mr. Pott was endowed with gifts of keen clinical observation and lucid exposition. In 1776 Mr. Pott studied cancer of the skin of the little "climbing boys" who swept the chimneys of England:

There is a disease as peculiar to a certain set of people, which has not, at least to my knowledge, been publicly noticed; I mean the chimney sweeper's cancer. It is a disease which always makes its first attack on, and its first appearance in, the inferior part of the scrotum; where it produces a superficial, painful, ragged, ill-looking sore, with hard and rising edges; the trade call it soot-wart. I never saw it under the age of puberty. The disease, in these people, seems to derive its origin from a lodgment of soot in the rugae of the scrotum.

Experimental Cancer Produced by Coal Tar

Katsusaburo Yamagiwa (1863–1930) was professor of pathology in the Imperial University, Tokyo. He suffered from tuberculosis of the larynx, which required him to refrain from speech for long periods, literally years on end.

Using a brush, Yamagiwa and his assistant Ichikawa (1916) painted both ears of rabbits with tar every 2–3 days for many months. Benign tumors (skin papillomas) and highly malignant carcinomas were evoked. Papillomas emerged after applying tar for 30–100 days. The carcinomas metastasized to regional lymph nodes. Yamagiwa and Ichikawa 1918 claimed that their results substantiated experimentally the hypothesis of Virchow, that chronic irritation is the cause of cancer.

The perseverance of the Japanese, succeeding where predecessors had failed, is noteworthy. Yamagiwa and Ichikawa 1916 remark, "Therefore our experimental design was moderately simple. But our experiment demanded extraordinary patience in order to carry it out year after year."

The success of Yamagiwa has been ascribed to an additional talent—proficiency in the art of calligraphy as practiced with the brush in Japan.

Carcinogenic Tars Produced in the Laboratory

Ernest Laurance Kennaway (1881–1958), a chemical pathologist, served as director of the Research Institute of the Royal Cancer Hospital (Free) from 1931 to 1946. Kennaway was already suffering from Parkinson's disease by 1929. A colleague writes, "Few knew him well; those who did had a great affection for him. He had a logical and orderly mind and an almost encyclopedic knowledge. Every morning there would be a daily routine painting his mice" (Cook, 1958). E. L. Kennaway and his disciples elucidated the field of hydrocarbon carcinogenesis, creating thereby one of the most noble chapters of science. The work began with homemade tars prepared in the chemical laboratory: "When isoprene is passed through a tube filled with hydrogen and heated to 820° C a mixture of compounds, chiefly aromatic, is formed; this material produces cancer in mice more rapidly and in larger percentage of animals than do many samples of coal tar" (Kennaway 1924).

The isoprene tar was applied semiweekly to a group of 100 mice beginning on 4 September 1923; the first tumor of the skin appeared after 18 applications 63 days later. The pyrolysis of acetylene was used similarly as a source of cancer-producing tars (Kennaway 1924).

Isolation of Pure Carcinogenic Hydrocarbons

Kennaway and his school demonstrated for the first time that malignant tumors similar to human cancers can be induced by the application of pure chemical compounds of known molecular structure to living cells. The Kennaway circle included many talented young organic chemists. Among these workers J. W. Cook (1900–) was the senior associate. Prodigious feats of chemical isolation, synthesis, proof of structure, and biological testing were accomplished by the group, but the initiative in the work was entirely due to Kennaway (Cook 1958).

The carcinogenic tars obtained from pyrolysis of acetylene or isoprene showed a pronounced and characteristic 3-band fluorescence evident at low dispersions; Hieger 1930 noticed that the spectrum of the carcinogenic mixtures resembled the strong fluorescence of benz[*a*]anthracene (I) (fig. 4.1; structural formulas of compounds are I–XII, fig. 4.1; XIII–XVII, fig. 4.2; and XVIII–XX, fig. 4.3).

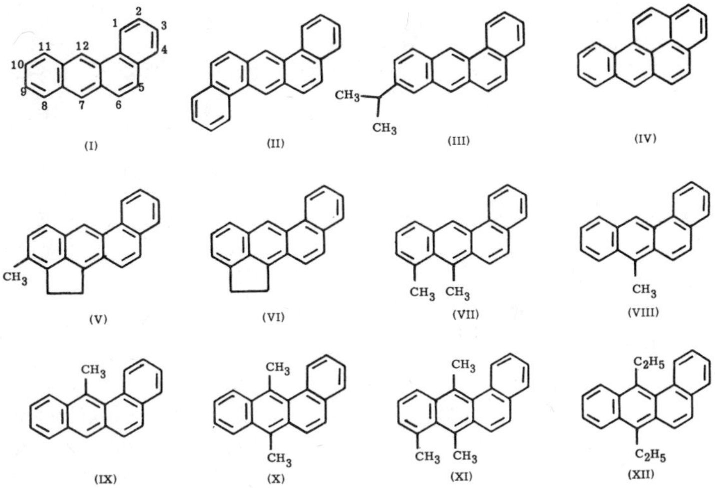

Fig. 4.1. The structural formulas of compounds I–XII.

Kennaway 1930 produced skin cancers in mice with a pure chemical compound; unfortunately the structural formula of the carcinogen was stated incorrectly (Cook et al. 1932).

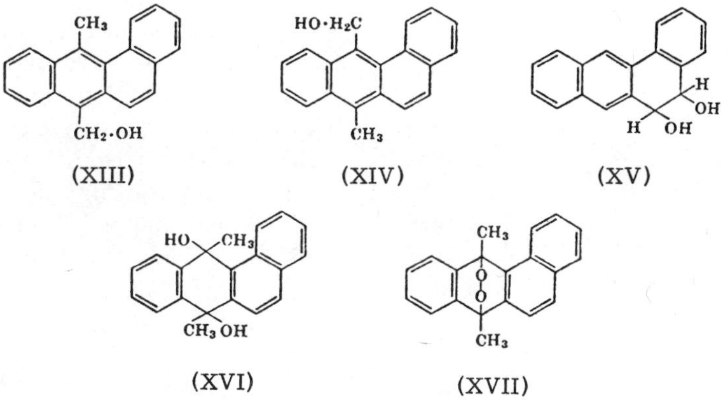

Fig. 4.2. The structural formulas of compounds XIII–XVII.

The voyages of discovery of progressively stronger pure carcinogenic hydrocarbons extended over six years culminating in the synthesis of 7,12-DMBA (Bachmann and Chemerda 1938).

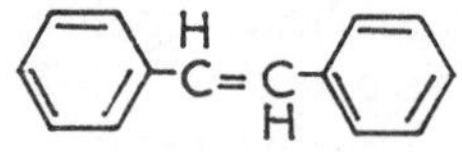

(XVIII)

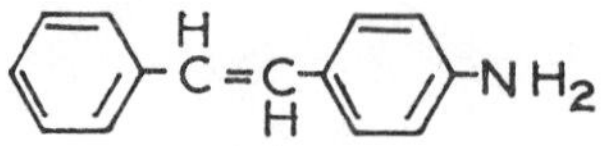

(XIX)

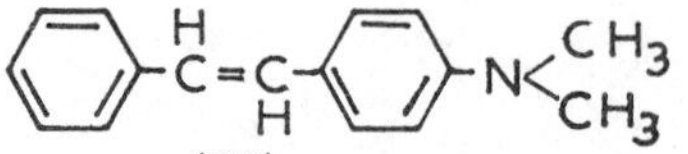

(XX)

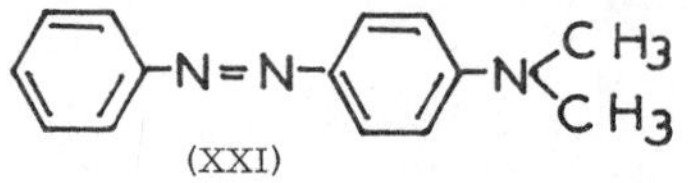

(XXI)

Fig. 4.3. The structural formulas of compounds XVIII–XXI.

The strong 3-band fluorescent spectrum of the carcinogenic tar mixtures led in 1932 to an examination of a large series of pure aromatic compounds related to benz[*a*]anthracene (BA). Two methods of biological testing were employed by Kennaway; first, solutions of the compounds were dropped from a pipette on the skin between the scapulae of stock mice to cause cutaneous papillomas and carcinomas; second, the compounds dissolved in lard were injected beneath the skin to evoke fibrosarcoma (Burrows, Hieger, and Kennaway 1932). Cook et al. 1932 found that one member of the BA series gave positive results; dibenz[*a,h*]anthracene (II) was the first pure hydrocarbon to be identified as a carcinogen; this compound had not been isolated from coal tars, but it had been synthesized by Clar.

Cook 1932 found that 9-isopropyl-BA (III) is carcinogenic. This observation showed that the pentacyclic structure of DBA (II) is not necessary in the production of cancer by compound III, which possesses only 4 rings.

In 1933, H. Wieland and Elizabeth Dane obtained a powerful carcinogen, 3-methylcholanthrene (V), from pyrolysis of a bile acid (Wieland and Dane 1933). Heinrich Wieland (1877–1957), an eminent student of biological oxidation-reduction, was professor of chemistry at Freiburg. Dehydro*nor*cholene (obtained by thermal destruction of 12-ketocholanic acid) was heated with Se at 150–250° C for 25 hr. After the distillation of impure organic material, 3-MC (V) was obtained by crystallization from benzene and acetic anhydride. The discovery of 3-MC had a profound effect on cancer research because it is a rather strong producer of cancer and because it was obtained from a natural product of animal cells rather than chimney soot.

By fractionation of two tons of coal tar pitch, Cook, Hewett, and Hieger 1933 obtained a crystalline material from which they isolated a strong carcinogenic hydrocarbon, benzo[a]pyrene (IV). Its solutions had the intense 3-band fluorescence of BA. Benzo[a]pyrene (IV) was the first pure carcinogenic substance isolated from coal tar.

Barry et al. 1935 synthesized 8-methyl-BA and found it to cause cancer. At that time it was surprising for the investigators to discover an active carcinogen that did not possess a substituent at position 9 of the benz[a]anthracene (I) structure.

In 1933 Fieser and Seligman (1935a, b) devised a total synthesis of 3-MC (V) and cholanthrene (VI). L. F. Fieser (1899–1977) was professor of chemistry at Harvard; Arnold M. Seligman (1912–76), then a medical student, was later professor of surgery at University of Maryland. From the carcinogenic activity of cholanthrene (VI) it was evident that the methyl group of 3-MC is not requisite for carcinogenesis. Sarcoma formed in 45 days after implanting crystals of 3-MC in mouse.

Fieser and Newman 1936 found that 7,8-DMBA (VII) was an active carcinogen; the cyclopenteno structure in cholanthrene was dispensable.

In 1937, 7-methyl-BA (VIII) was synthesized by two groups (Bachmann et al. 1937; Fieser and Hershberg 1937) and found to be an active carcinogen. All of the monomethyl isomers of BA have been synthesized; of these compounds 7-MBA (VIII) is the most powerful carcinogen, followed in activity by 12-MBA (IX) (Fieser and Hershberg 1937; Badger et al. 1940).

The year 1938 was the year of synthesis of 7,12-DMBA (X) and 7,8,12-TMBA (XI). In one of the most elegant, hence the most useful, contributions to cancer research Bachmann and Chemerda 1938 described the synthesis of three new polycyclic aromatic hydrocarbons: 7,12-dimethyl-, 7,12-diethyl-, and 7,8,12-trimethylbenz[a]anthracene. Although 7,12-DMBA and 7,8,12-TMBA are the most potent chemical carcinogens, 7,12-diethylbenz[a]anthracene (XII) does not produce cancer. The carcinogen 7,12-DMBA was prepared in four steps from benz[a]anthracene-7,12-quinone; the yield was 96%.

Werner Bachmann (1901–51) had studied as a postdoctoral fellow in the Kennaway laboratory; later he was professor of chemistry at the University of Michigan, Ann Arbor. He was an inspired teacher and a creative research chemist who had a keen and intuitive insight for organic reactions. He recognized the importance of the perfection of methods in solving difficult problems.

Bachmann and the Kennaways 1938 tested two of the new compounds (X and XI) for cancer-producing activity in London and found them to be exceedingly potent; one drop of 0.3% solution of the compound in benzene was applied twice weekly to the interscapular skin of stock mice. Two of the most active carcinogens, BP and 3-MC, were assayed concurrently; both of these control compounds elicited tumors of which the majority began to appear after 100 days and 75 days, respectively. Both 7,12-DMBA and 7,8,12-TMBA were found to be highly carcinogenic; when applied to mice in the usual way, skin tumors appeared in many mice by day 35. In the mice 7,12-DMBA showed unusual results: *i*, multiplicity of tumors to an extent greater than had been produced hitherto by other compounds, *ii*, epilation over an especially large area, and *iii*, extreme rapidity of carcinogenesis.

Whereas 7-methyl-BA and 7-ethyl-BA are carcinogens, Shear and Leiter 1940 discovered that 7-propyl-BA and 7-butyl-BA do not cause cancer. Since 1938 no chemical compound has been found to equal in intensity the carcinogenic effects of 7,12-DMBA and 7,8,12-TMBA.

Fluorine substitution in carcinogenic hydrocarbons is informative concerning the molecular action of carcinogens. F is a small atom that does not deform the geometry of the molecule, forms strong covalent F-C bonds, and withdraws electrons from the ring structure. Miller and Miller 1960, 1963 found that fluorine substitution in 7-MBA to form 5F-7-MBA virtually abolished its cancer-producing activity, whereas 6F-7-MBA is a strong carcinogen. Bergmann, Blum, and Haddow 1963 found that 5F-7,12-DMBA is devoid of carcinogenicity. We have observed that 1F-7,12-DMBA and 2F-7,12-DMBA do not elicit sarcoma.

Metabolism of 7,12-DMBA

The metabolism of 7,12-DMBA in the rat was investigated in the classic study of Boyland and Sims 1965. The metabolic pathways consist primarily of oxygenation of the methyl groups and to a small extent of the ring structure. The main products of metabolism of 7,12-DMBA by rat liver homogenates are the isomeric monohydroxymethyl derivatives: 7-hydroxymethyl-12-methyl-BA (XIII) and 7-methyl-12-hydroxymethyl-BA (XIV). Small amounts of phenols, diols, epoxides, and dihydrodihydroxy compounds (XV and XVI) as well as 7,12-*epi*dioxy-7,12-DMBA (XVII) were detected. All of the metabolic products arise from the action of mixed function oxidases (p. 146) in microsomes, primarily of the liver. Similarly, monohydroxymethyl derivatives are products of the hydroxylation of 7,12-DMBA in the ascorbic acid-Fe^{2+}-oxygen hydroxylating system of Udenfriend et al. 1954. Other dihydrodiols of many sorts involving the ring structure have been found in small amounts (Yang and Dower 1975).

Pretreatment of rats with aromatic compounds including 3-MC and small amounts of 7,12-DMBA itself protects the animals from adrenal necrosis caused by 7,12-DMBA by inducing detoxifying enzymes in hepatic microsomes. Yang and Dower 1975 showed that the induced microsomes efficiently metabolize 7,12-DMBA, both in the ring positions and in the production of monohydroxymethyl derivatives.

Aromatic Amines: Anesthetic Carcinogens

The aromatic amines differ from the polycyclic aromatic hydrocarbons in three important respects: first, they have a propensity for inducing tumors in the liver; second, they oxidize hemoglobin to methemoglobin; and, third, some of them are anesthetic agents that induce sleep while causing cancer. Among the compounds which, when fed, oxidize Hb to MetHb are 1-naphthylamine, 2-naphthylamine, 4-aminodiphenyl, and 4-aminostilbene.

We have observed that the feeding of large quantities of the carcinogenic aromatic amines to rats produces ataxia and deep sleep of some hours duration. The compounds were dissolved in sesame oil and administered by gastric tube. Sleep-producing doses of the aromatic amines were 100 mg of 2-naphthylamine, 150 mg of 2-aminophenanthrene, 75 mg of 4-aminostilbene, 50 mg of 4-aminodiphenyl. All of these compounds are carcinogens.

Aminostilbenes. The study of compounds in this series by Haddow et al. 1948 is a classic investigation which arose from Haddow's discovery that an unusually marked inhibition of the rapidly growing Walker carcinoma occurred in rats injected with 4-aminostilbene (4-AS) and 4-dimethylaminostilbene (4-DMAS). The tumor inhibitory action of these compounds was less pronounced in mice.

Stilbene (XVIII) is not toxic and does not evoke cancer, whereas the addition of strongly basic substituents to form 4-AS (XIX) and 4-DMAS (XX) and congeners results in highly toxic compounds that are powerful carcinogens. In toxicity studies in our laboratory, rats were given a single feeding of 4-DMAS dissolved in sesame oil; the dose causing death of half of the animals in 21 days (LD_{50}) was 90 mg/kg. In doses of 200–250 mg in rat, 4-AS and 4-DMAS produce gastric hemorrhages and hematuria (Haddow et al. 1948).

Dissolved in sesame oil and injected in rats, 4-AS and certain congeners gave rise to local and distant tumors. Of 72 rats injected with 4-amino-, 4-acetamido-, 4-dimethylamino-, or 4-diethylaminostilbene, 23 animals developed a total of 8 local sarcomas and 30 distant tumors, mostly carcinomas, involving ear duct, mammary gland, and liver (cholangiomas).

Aminoazo Dyes. Sasaki and Yoshida 1935 discovered that the addition of *o*-aminoazotoluol (AAT) to the diet of rats produced tumors of the liver. The earliest hepatoma was found after feeding the dye for 196 days and without exception every rat fed for 255–300 days had liver tumors. Kinosita 1936 found that 4-dimethylaminoazobenzene (DAB, XXI) was more active as a hepatic carcinogen than AAT was. DAB is usually fed to rats at a level of 0.06% in the diet; under appropriate conditions there is a high incidence of liver tumors in 120–160 days (Miller and Miller 1953). The aminoazo dyes do not evoke distant tumors.

2-Acetylaminofluorene. Wilson, DeEds, and Cox 1941 found that a powerful insecticide, 2-acetylaminofluorene is an active carcinogen; they incorporated this compound at a level of 0.03% in the ration of rats which was fed to rats for 95 or more days. Of 39 rats 19 developed tumors. Many rats developed liver and bladder tumors and mammary cancers. Leukemia was elicited in two animals.

5 Induction of Sarcoma

There is only one unambiguous experimental method to determine carcinogenicity; it is to ascertain if your compound produces cancer in animals. Guinea pig is resistant but mouse and rat are extremely susceptible to cancer-producing chemical compounds. The induction of sarcoma of fibroblasts in rat or mouse is a method of extreme simplicity, economical of resource, space, and compound; sarcoma is detected in 1–9 months and the results are unequivocal.

In postembryonic life, fibroblasts have a unique lability of phenotype; the cell's program can be altered readily (p. 13). This remarkable mutability is closely related to the vulnerability of the genome. In living animals fibroblasts become sarcoma cells after exposure to viruses, irradiation or aromatic hydrocarbons. With respect to viruses, it is noteworthy that only the Rous sarcoma viruses will transform fibroblasts into sarcoma cells at the point of local injection in living animals. Nö other virus elicits sarcoma at the injection site.

Radiation-Induced Fibrosarcoma

The special vulnerability of fibroblasts to x-irradiation was demonstrated in two strains of rat, S-D (albino) and L-E (piebald), by Huggins and Fukunishi 1963a. Sublethal, total-body irradiation preferentially injured three classes of cells, marrow, mammary glands, and fibroblasts. X-irradiation induced two sorts of malignant disease, mammary carcinoma (p. 74) and sarcoma of fibroblasts. There were no more. Quite remarkably, leukemia was not observed. Sarcoma usually was periosteal but sarcomas of the mesentery also were found.

Method 5.1: Radiation-Induced Sarcoma

For all irradiations (Huggins and Fukunishi 1963a) we used a 250-kvp x-ray machine, operating at 30 ma, with a 0.5 mm Cu and 1 mm Al filter, HVL 1.5 mm Cu, and FSD of 99 cm. The dose rate "free in air," determined by a 250 r capacity Victoreen, was 27.7 r/min at a point corresponding to the midpoint of the animals. The rats were placed in individual compartments, with a perforated aluminum lid, on a turntable. Twelve rats were irradiated simultaneously. A total dose of 400r was delivered in a single exposure and the day of irradiation is designated day 0.

Albino Rat. A grand total of 146 female S-D rats survived 6+ months after a single total-body irradiation with 400r of x-rays. The incidence of neoplasms was mammary cancer in 36 rats (24.7%) and sarcoma in 8 rats (5.5%).

Piebald Rat. In all, 71 female L-E rats survived for 6 months after a single total-body irradiation (400r). The incidence of neoplasms was sarcoma in 2 rats (2.8%) but no mammary cancer.

Not all of the many millions of mammary cells or fibroblasts developed carcinomas or sarcomas—only a few tumors arose and these were found in only a small proportion of the irradiated animals. It would appear that the cancerous transformation of radiation is restricted to a small number of cells that are vulnerable during 14.4 min required to deliver 400r of total-body irradiation during our experiment.

Sarcoma Induced Locally by Hydrocarbons

Three tissues of the rat and mouse are exceptionally vulnerable to the induction of malignant tumors by carcinogenic polycyclic aromatic hydrocarbons, or aromatic amines. The cancer-prone cells are the mammary acini, hemapoietic stem-cells, and fibroblasts. Both classes of compounds elicit a similar pattern of tumors in genetically susceptible rodents and these selectively evoked neoplasms become evident rapidly and in profusion. The patterns are consistent for rat and for mouse, but these species differ somewhat with regard to the types of tumors that are elicited.

Different methods are required to elicit cancer in the various susceptible tissues by means of the most potent carcinogenic compounds. In the case of the mammary tubules, a single flash exposure to 7,12-DMBA or 7,8,12-TMBA, achieved by an intravenous injection, elicits mammary cancer in nearly every animal (p. 81). A solitary injection seldom elicits leukemia; in the case of hematopoietic stem-cells multiple doses (p. 119) of potent hydrocarbons are necessary to produce leukemia in rat and mouse.

A single intravenous injection of a carcinogenic hydrocarbon never elicits sarcoma; the production of sarcoma requires prolonged contact (p. 71) between potent carcinogen and responsive cell because mitosis is sluggish in the cells of the connective tissue. Mitotic cell division is mandatory for the production of cancer.

In the classical induction of sarcoma by polycyclic aromatic hydrocarbons or aromatic amines, the compound dissolved in an organic solvent or vegetable oil is injected intramuscularly or subcutaneously in rat or mouse. The method is convenient and a valuable indicator of carcinogenicity; it is especially useful when the total amount of available compound is small, say 5–10 mg. Burrows, Hieger, and Kennaway 1932 found that subcutaneous injection of DBA in lard produced spindle cell sarcomas in 31/93 mice and 15/67 rats; the sarcomas were readily transplantable for many generations.

Proposition 1: Induction of Sarcoma

Long-Evans rat, aged 25 days, injected in thigh muscle with 2.5 mg of 3-methylcholanthrene dissolved in 0.5 ml of sesame oil, will develop fibrosarcoma at the injection site within 120 days.

A study of structure-activity of closely related polycyclic aromatic hydrocarbons was carried out by Huggins, Pataki, and Harvey 1967. The motivation was a fascinating problem: in rat 7,12-dimethylbenz[*a*]anthracene is the most potent of the chemical carcinogens, whereas 7,12-diethylbenz[*a*]anthracene does not elicit malignant tumors in the rat or any other species. It is evident that profound differences in carcinogenicity accompany trivial structural changes in polynuclear aromatic hydrocarbons. Molecular thickness of the carcinogen was found to be a determinant in carcinogenicity.

The experiments were initiated because we had found striking differences in the pharmacology of 7,12-dialkyl derivatives of BA. Under stated conditions spectacular effects in the rat are brought about invariably by a single large dose of 7,12-DMBA. These include induction of mammary cancer, massive and selective destruction of certain layers of adrenal cortex and testis, and great toxicity in rat though not in mouse or ground squirrel, in which species 7,12-DMBA is devoid of toxicity (Huggins, Ford, and Jensen 1965).

A series of small alkyl and alkoxyl derivatives of BA was assayed for the ability to induce sarcoma (see method 5.2) following intramuscular injection (Huggins, Pataki, and Harvey 1967). Our samples of sesame oil (used as solvent) or of BA did not elicit sarcoma. The ring system must be more reactive than BA is. The minimum basicity for carcinogenicity was provided by a single methyl group, which, added to BA, created certain highly carcinogenic compounds.

Method 5.2: Induction of Sarcoma by Lipid-Soluble Compounds

The compound was dissolved, 0.5% w/v, in sesame oil by heating for ~ 1 hr in an oven at 100° C. The recipients were male L-E rats, usually aged 25 days, 6 to 8 in each set; each rat was injected (day 0) with 0.5 ml of the solution (2.5 mg of compound) in thigh muscle of each leg. Necropsy was performed when a large firm lump with a characteristic firm consistency was detected; the experiment was terminated on day 270. At necropsy a pool of oil was always found marking the injection site. The sarcoma is transplanted by inserting 50–100 mg of the neoplasm subcutaneously in an allogeneic recipient.

Monoalkyl Substitution of BA. The site of a methyl substituent of the BA molecule is decisive in its importance in rendering the inactive molecule carcinogenic. Monomethyl derivatives of BA had been tested in earlier studies. In mice, Badger et al. 1942 found only three of the derivatives were strong carcinogens; these were 7-methyl-, 8-methyl-, and 12-methyl-BA. In rat, Dunning and Curtis 1960 found that four of these compounds were strong carcinogens; these were 6-, 7-, 8-, and 12-methyl-BA. Bergmann 1942 found that five monomethyl derivatives of BA were active carcinogens, namely, 6-, 7-, 8-, 9-, and 12-methyl-BA.

Huggins, Pataki, and Harvey 1967 found that four monomethyl derivatives of BA elicited sarcoma in the rat; the carcinogens were 6-, 7-, 8-, and 12-methyl-BA. All of the monomethyl-substituted derivatives of BA had a significant association with cellular constituents since a single feeding of 10 mg of the 12 compounds, given one at a time, greatly induced the synthesis of the soluble drug-metabolizing hepatic enzyme, menadione reductase (p. 147). But molecular sites 6, 7, 8, 9, and 12 in the BA molecule, located in or near the *meso* position, form an intramolecular triangle of outstanding importance in creating highly powerful carcinogenic agents. It is the fiery trigon.

The derivatives 7-methoxy-BA, 7-ethyl-BA, and 12-ethyl-BA were feeble carcinogens which induced sarcoma in ~ 5% of the rats; 7-propyl-BA was inactive.

The carcinogenic influence of the alkyl groups in the fiery triangle (fig. 5.1) of BA, related to the *meso* position, is attributed to electronic factors. The small alkyl groups have a high ionization potential consistent with resonance interactions

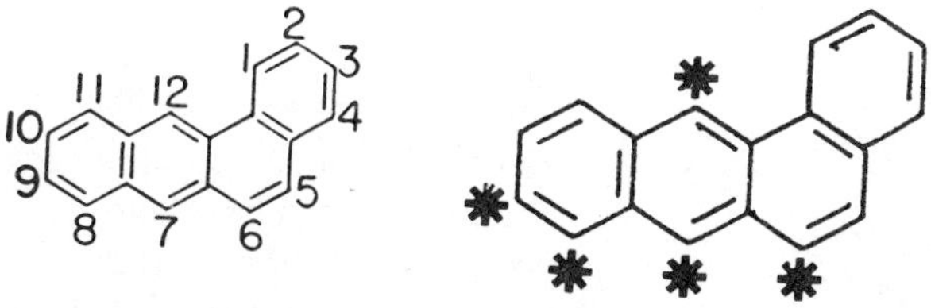

Fig. 5.1. The numbering system of benz[a]anthracene is shown. Introduction of one or more small alkyl groups at special sites (*) converts the inactive molecule (BA) into a carcinogen.

of hyperconjugation and their position in the favored triangle is advantageous for association during the stage of replication of DNA when the underlying purine-pyrimidine base pairs separate.

Dialkyl Substitution of Benz[a]anthracene. An experiment was designed to investigate the influence of molecular thickness of derivatives of BA on carcinogenicity. A series of 7,12-dialkyl-benz[a]anthracenes was synthesized comprising the four possible combinations (table 5.1) of methyl-ethyl groups in the *meso* position of BA (Huggins, Pataki, and Harvey 1967). One member of the group, 7,12-diethylbenz[a]anthracene, was inactive in eliciting sarcoma, whereas three members of the series were active carcinogens. The active compounds that produced sarcoma are given in order of decreasing carcinogenicity: 7,12-DMBA = 7-ethyl-12-methyl-BA > 7-methyl-12-ethyl-BA.

Table 5.1   Sarcoma Induced by Dialkyl Derivatives of Benz[a]anthracene

Compound	Number of rats	Number with sarcoma	Detection of Sarcoma (days)	
			Range	Mean
7,12-DMBA	20	20	67–116	87 ± 20
7-Et-12-MBA	15	15	68– 95	84 ± 10
7-Me-12-Et-BA	16	11	107–257	155 ± 55
7,12-DEBA	24	0	—	—

NOTE: Male rats, age 25 days, were injected intramuscularly in each leg with 0.5 ml of sesame oil containing 2.5 mg of hydrocarbon. The animals were sacrificed after 9 months or when sarcomas were detected earlier. Means with standard deviation ± are given.

None of these congeners is flat. The ring system of each is slightly buckled, and, additionally, three of the compounds possess bulky groups. The carcinogens 7-ethyl-12-methyl-BA and 7-methyl-12-ethyl-BA have a large substituent but only on one surface of the molecule. The inactive compound 7,12-DEBA has thick alkyl groups on both its top and bottom surfaces.

Steric relationships are the most reasonable explanation for the differences in carcinogenicity of the methyl-ethyl *meso* substituted derivatives of BA. It would appear that face-to-face association of some critical component of the cell is required to elicit the specific mutation of cancer. The association still can occur provided one surface, top or bottom, does not exceed 4 Å in height. But when the height of *both* the top and bottom surfaces of the molecule exceeds 4 Å (as in 7,12-DEBA) close association cannot take place in the cell, and the compound is inactive as a carcinogen.

Sarcoma Induced Remotely by 3-MC

When groups of rats repeatedly were fed the strong carcinogen 3-MC and injected concurrently with sesame oil or saline in the scruff of the neck or leg, sarcoma developed in high yields in the injection sites (Huggins and Grand 1963).

The experimental animals were female S-D rats, age 50 days. Sesame oil was purified by molecular distillation; 3-MC was recrystallized from benzene and ether. Sesame oil or 0.15 M NaCl was injected subcutaneously; 3-MC, 10 mg, dissolved in sesame oil was fed by gastric intubation. The feedings of 3-MC and the injections were given 6 days each week.

There were two groups of controls: in one sesame oil was injected but 3-MC was not fed and in the other 3-MC was fed but injections were not given. Sarcoma did not develop in either group.

Sesame oil (0.2 ml daily) was injected for 100 days alternately in right and left legs of 14 rats fed 3-MC (10 mg daily) for the first 50 days of the experiment. Fibrosarcoma was found in the legs of every rat in 98 to 203 days. In a similar experiment, except that sesame oil was injected into the scruff, sarcoma (fig. 5.2) arose in the neck of 8 of 10 rats. Four of the sarcomas were excised and 50–100 mg fragments were transplanted subcutaneously in female rats age 46 days; "takes," with subsequent vigorous growth of the sarcoma, occurred in 14 of 35 transplants of this type, and the histologic appearance of the transplant was fibrosarcoma resembling the original tumor.

Sodium chloride, 0.5 ml, was injected repeatedly in the neck of 12 rats that were fed 3-MC concurrently; sarcomas developed in the scruff of 3 rats in 162–203 days.

The experiments prove that repeated trauma can cause the localization of circulating carcinogens and thereby elicit sarcoma at the site of injury. Bryan and Shimkin 1943 found that the subcutaneous injection of 21 μg of 3-MC elicited sarcoma in 50% of C3H mice.

Intraperitoneal Administration of 7,12-DMBA

In albino rats an intraperitoneal injection of a lipid emulsion of 7,12-DMBA caused no fatalities and failed to produce sarcomas of the peritoneum, but mammary carcinoma (p. 82) arose with high frequency (Huggins and Fukunishi 1963*b*). This effect was manifest whether newborn or adult rats were the recipients of the homogenized carcinogen. But peritoneal sarcomas developed in high yield when a compressed pellet of 7,12-DMBA was deposited surgically to remain in the peritoneal cavity of the young adult rats.

Newborn Rats. The toxicity (LD_{50}) of homogenized 7,12-DMBA was determined. Newborn rats in our colony weighing 6 gm were injected intraperitoneally with an emulsion of 7,12-DMBA, 0.5% w/v, and the amount of hydrocarbon causing the death of half of the animals within 21 days was determined; the LD_{50} was 50 mg/kg (0.3 mg per rat).

At birth, 15 female and 18 male rats were injected with an emulsion containing 7,12-DMBA, 0.25 mg, and the yield of tumors was determined; the experiment terminated on day 180. The incidence of mammary carcinoma was 8 females and no males. Peritoneal sarcomas did not form in any rat.

A difference in genetic constitution is already apparent at birth in the mammary glands of newborn S-D and L-E rats vis-à-vis tumor formation in the mammary gland after a single intraperitoneal injection of 7,12-DMBA. Benign mammary fibroadenomas were evoked in high and similar incidence in both strains. The racial difference concerns mammary cancer; carcinoma of the breast occurred in high incidence in S-D rats, whereas in L-E rats the incidence was 5.1%.

Young Adult Rats. A single intraperitoneal injection of the emulsion containing 7,12-DMBA induced mammary cancer preferentially within 2 months in all young adult S-D female rats. Ten female S-D rats, age 50 days, were injected intraperitoneally with emulsified 7,12-DMBA, 5 mg; mammary cancer developed in every rat in 36 to 56 days; peritoneal sarcomas did not develop. Quantitatively the intraperitoneal injection of an emulsion of 7,12-DMBA is similar to intravenous injection in its high efficiency in evoking mammary tumors (Huggins and Fukunishi 1963*b*).

Intraperitoneal Pellets of 7,12-DMBA. An observation of interest in the present work concerned the peritoneal tumors; it is remarkable that none occurred after injection of the emulsion of 7,12-DMBA into the peritoneal cavity. Yet the peritoneal cells are not insusceptible to the carcinogenic effects of this hydrocarbon; a compressed pellet of 7,12-DMBA deposited in

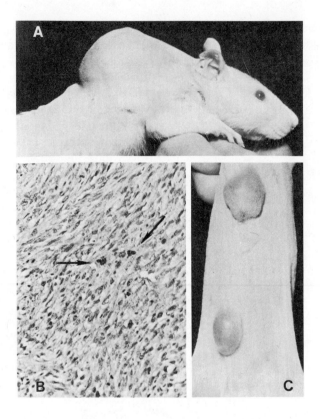

Fig. 5.2. *A*. Sarcoma in neck of a rat 178 days following the commencement of daily feeding of 3-methylcholanthrene, 10 mg, and the daily injection of sesame oil, 0.2 ml. The injections lasted 50 days. *B*. Photomicrograph of histological section of sarcoma; the arrows point to mitotic figures. *C*. Sarcomas arose from two fragments of a tumor 20 days after transplantation subcutaneously into female rats age 46 days.

the peritoneal cavity evoked tumors of the peritoneum in most rats. It would appear that not every cell of the rat is susceptible at all times to malignancy after contact with carcinogenic hydrocarbons and that an emulsion of 7,12-DMBA disappears from the peritoneal cavity before adequate contact with a cell in a state susceptible to the malignant transformation. In this regard, a pellet in prolonged contact with peritoneal cells sooner or later finds cells prone to sarcoma formation.

A sterile compressed pellet of 7,12-DMBA (15–25 mg) was deposited surgically in the peritoneal cavity of 17 S-D female rats, age 50 days, and the animals were observed for 7 months. At autopsy the pellet was found free-floating in 2 rats and it was encapsulated in the others. Fourteen of the rats developed tumors at the site of encapsulation: spindle-cell sarcoma 11 and mesothelioma 3. Two rats with peritoneal sarcoma developed mammary cancer.

6 Induction of Mammary Cancer in Rat

There are two ways to induce cancer in the breast in the rat. Mammary cancer forms readily and grows rapidly in young female rats of susceptible strains given a solitary dose of (*i*) ionizing radiation or (*ii*) the most powerful carcinogenic hydrocarbons. Both procedures are exceedingly easy to carry out. The hydrocarbons are more efficacious qua carcinogens than radiation is.

The mammary acini of young female albino rats are foremost among the cells of living creatures in their susceptibility to the induction of cancer by chemical substances or irradiation. Mammary adenocarcinoma is evoked selectively and regularly by a flash exposure of the cells to carcinogens; this is accomplished by a single pulse-injection in a vein of lipid emulsions of the most potent cancer-producing aromatic hydrocarbons or aromatic amines. It can also be achieved by a single feeding of a massive but generally tolerable amount of the carcinogenic compounds. These procedures mimic ionizing radiation in damaging selectively certain chromosomes during replication. Under stipulated conditions most of the mammary cancers become evident in the living animal in 3–9 weeks. The cancer-inductive effect of the aromatics is one of the most dramatic displays in science.

Proposition 2: Induction of Mammary Cancer

Under stated conditions every intact female rat of Sprague-Dawley strain fed a single meal of 20 mg of 7,12-dimethylbenz[a]anthracene (∼130 mg/kg) in 2 ml of sesame oil at age 50 days will develop mammary adenocarcinoma or leukemia.

The stipulated conditions (Huggins 1965) include nine parameters: the nature and dosage of the carcinogen and the species, strain, sex, age, and hormonal status of the recipient; in addition, the rats must be free from pneumonitis and have had no contact with cancer protective substances (p. 152). Pneumonitis is prevented by painfully clean, hygienic conditions in the housing of the colony.

Each of 115 female S-D rats, age 50 days, was fed a single meal of 20 mg of 7,12-DMBA; there were 5 deaths before day 20. The incidence of neoplasms in 110 effective rats was 109 with mammary carcinoma and 1 with leukemia. As controls 164 female S-D rats, virgin and untreated, were observed for 6 months; spontaneous mammary carcinoma was observed in 2 rats (1.2%) and lymphosarcoma in 1 rat.

Mammary acini of Sprague-Dawley and Wistar rats (both strains are albino) are immensely susceptible, whereas the mammary glands of rats of Long-Evans (pigmented) strain are resistant to a single onslaught of the carcinogenic agents. Susceptibility to mammary cancer is a function of the genetic constitution of the animals but *resistance of the mammary glands of the L-E strain can be abolished by a set of multiple doses of aromatic hydrocarbons*; now the L-E strain becomes highly susceptible to development of mammary cancer.

Radiation-Induced Mammary Carcinoma

In the rat a single exposure to a sublethal dose of total-body irradiation results in the preferential induction of mammary cancer and fibrosarcoma. When given a single dose of the carcinogenic hydrocarbons, young female albino rats of S-D strain are susceptible, whereas rats of L-E strain are resistant to mammary cancer; the same pattern occurs when mammary cancer is induced by radiation. Radiation-induced fibrosarcoma (p. 66) developed in both S-D and L-E strains, males and females, of all ages; cancer of the breast arose only in S-D stock.

In the experiments of Hamilton, Durbin, and Parrott 1954, a considerable proportion (40%) of female S-D rats, age 55 days, developed mammary cancer after a single pulse-injection of [211]Astatine, an α-particle emitter; this isotope, also known as *eka*-iodine, destroys the thyroid glands of the recipients.

Shellabarger et al. 1957 found that 42% of a series of female S-D rats, age 40 days, developed mammary adenocarcinoma after total-body x-irradiation (200–400r) with a ^{60}Co irradiator.

In the study of Cronkite et al. 1960, it was found that many S-D females developed mammary tumors, benign and malignant, within 10 months after exposure to a single dose (400r) of total-body x-irradiation. The first tumor was detected 41 days after irradiation. Removal of the ovaries, before or after total-body irradiation, reduced but did not eliminate the incidence of cancer of the breast. The mammary tumors were carcinoma, fibroadenoma, and fibrosarcoma (Bond et al. 1959). Few tumors were elicited other than those in the mammary glands. Young female rats were more vulnerable than older females were. The incidence of mammary tumors was 2% of nonexposed controls, 79% with irradiation at age 40 days, and 25% with irradiation at age 120 days. With half-body exposure approximately one-half the total number of neoplasms found after total-body irradiation was observed; direct radiation injury to the mammary glands is necessary for irradiation-induced neoplasia.

Mammary Cancer Elicited by X-Irradiation. Young adult female rats of two strains were subjected to a heavy dose (400r) of total-body x-irradiation (method 5.1) and observed for 6–12 months thereafter (Huggins and Fukunishi 1963*a*). Only two sorts of malignant tumors were produced—sarcoma (p. 65) and mammary carcinoma.

1. In the L-E strain, 33 female piebald rats irradiated on a single occasion at age 52 days survived for 6+ months; the incidence of neoplasms was no mammary carcinoma and 2 rats (6%) with sarcoma.

2. In the S-D strain, 74 female albino rats irradiated on a single occasion at age 52 days survived 6 months thereafter; the incidence of neoplasms was 22 with mammary carcinoma (30%) and 3 with sarcoma (4%). Mammary cancers were detected at 25–133 days (mean 54.9 ± 29 days).

Sublethal irradiation caused severe damage to the marrow, whereas pituitary and ovary were spared from injury. The irradiation caused a precipitous decline (fig. 6.1) in the number of leukocytes in venous blood with severe lymphocyte depression; the most profound leukopenia was reached on day 4 after the irradiation; later there was a return to preradiation levels.

In one set of experiments, 15 S-D female rats survived for a year after x-irradiation (400r) at age 52 days; vaginal cytology was examined (method 3.1) daily in every animal. In the irradiated group estrus was present on an average of one cycle every 4.95 days. In nonirradiated controls estrus occurred on an average of every 4.15 days.

Mammary carcinomas in S-D rats, whether induced by irradiation or by polycyclic aromatic hydrocarbons, shared the following qualities: similar histological appearance; similar regressive properties after ovariex; and similar content of five dehydrogenases—glucose-6-phosphate, 6-phosphogluconic, isocitric, lactic, and malic (Huggins and Fukunishi 1963*a*).

Hydrocarbon-Induced Mammary Carcinoma

2-Acetylaminofluorene. Wilson, DeEds, and Cox 1941 were the first to observe that distant tumors arose following the in-

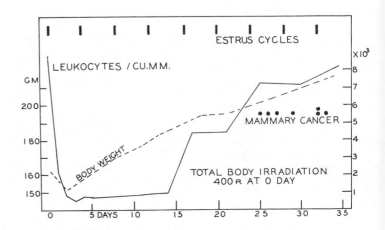

Fig. 6.1. Following a single total-body irradiation at age 52 days (day 0) there was a severe leukopenia and yet estrus cycles were retained in rats free from fatal radiation sickness. The day of detection of mammary cancer is indicated.

corporation of AAF in a ration that was fed ad libitum to rats for prolonged periods; tumors arose in liver, bladder, mammary glands, and other organs. The cancer-producing effect of AAF in the diet was confirmed by Bielschowsky 1944. These experiments established the importance of the gastrointestinal tract as a portal of entry for mammary carcinogens.

In an experiment in which AAF (daily dose $\sim$ 4 mg) was mixed in the ration fed to young female rats of two strains for 25 weeks, it was found that mammary cancer was elicited in high incidence (60%) in albino rats of the Wistar strain and in low incidence (4%) in pigmented rats (Bielschowsky 1946).

The induction of cancer by feeding carcinogens in the ration is semiquantitative and wasteful of compounds; this method has become outmoded.

Miller and Miller 1962 designate N-hydroxy-2-acetylaminofluorene a "proximate" carcinogen; when 2 mg of this compound in aqueous suspension was injected intraperitoneally in weanling rats, the incidence of mammary cancer was 50% at 15 weeks. The incidence of mammary cancers was not high and the rate of development of the tumors was slow.

3-Methylcholanthrene. In studying carcinogenesis, Maisin and Coolen 1936 painted the skin of mice with a solution of 3-MC for many months and observed that, in addition to producing cancer of the skin, mammary cancer arose in 18% of the animals. Englebreth-Holm 1941 repeated the experiment and found that mammary cancer formed only in females, whereas the male mice were not susceptible.

Shay et al. 1949 carried out admirable studies whose primary purpose was the experimental production of cancer of the gastric glands by repeated instillation of a solution of 3-MC in rat's stomach. Cancer of the stomach did not arise, but remarkably cancers of the mammary gland did. By means of gastric intubation Shay et al. 1949, 1951 and Shay, Harris, and Gruenstein 1952 fed rats of the Wistar strain a fixed daily dose (2 mg) of 3-MC six times each week for many months. Mammary carcinoma was elicited in high incidence in intact females, whereas significantly fewer mammary neoplasms developed in males or in castrate females treated in the same fashion. In the males, some of the tumors were fibrosarcomas of the breast or mesentery. In the intact females mammary cancer was detected after 4 months and the incidence of mammary tumors after one year was 100%; a long time was required for the tumors to become manifest. The method was laborious and potentially dangerous since daily handling of the carcinogen was carried on for months.

In the experiments of Huggins, Briziarelli, and Sutton 1959, 3-MC (10 mg) was fed by stomach tube to young S-D female rats for 7 weeks according to various schedules. All of the rats developed mammary cancer regardless of feeding 1 day or 6 days each week (table 6.1).

Table 6.1   Influence of Frequency of Feeding 3-MC on
                                 Induction of Mammary Cancer

Frequency of tube-feeding (days each week)	Appearance of mammary cancer (in days)		
	Range	Median	Mean
1	49–100	69	67.3
2	37– 85	52	58.4
3	44– 56	51	50.1
4	44– 64	56	55.9
5	44– 64	51	54.1
6	37– 58	44	47.8

NOTE: 3-MC (10 mg) was administered by gastric intubation to S-D females for 7 weeks beginning at age 50 days with 10 rats in each group; *mammary carcinoma developed in every rat.*

A single feeding by gastric tube (method 6.1) of 3-MC (660 mg/kg) to S-D females, age 50 days, was lethal for ~ 10% of the rats; in most instances the cause of death was aplastic anemia. In 100 consecutive survivors the incidence of neoplasms was 100% for mammary carcinoma and 2% for squamous carcinoma of ear glands. No tumors arose in 20 male rats treated in the same way as the aforementioned females. This experiment showed that *a single meal can initiate cancer of the breast.* The female rats lost weight ($\sim$ 13% of starting values) for 72 hr but gained on day 4; diarrhea was absent. Mammary cancer was detected in 46–72 days; the mean was 60.2 $\pm$ 9 days (table 6.2). The mean number of active centers (mammary cancers found in the gross at necropsy) was 2.3. The induction of mammary cancer was satisfactory but the tumors were slow in becoming manifest.

Table 6.2   Mammary Cancer Evoked in Female S-D Rats by a Solitary Feeding of 3-MC or 7,12-DMBA

				Mammary cancer detected		
Compound	Dose (mg)	Number of rats	Early deaths	Number of rats	Range (days)	Mean (days)
3-MC	100	10	1	9	46–72	60.2 $\pm$ 9*
7,12-DMBA	20	9	1	8	24–59	42.8 $\pm$ 10*

NOTE: The animals received the compound by tube-feeding at age 50 days. Means with standard deviation $\pm$ are given.
*Significant difference: $P < 0.005$.

As a causative agent for the induction of mammary cancer, 3-MC is advantageous insofar as it is rather nontoxic when multiple feedings are given. A disadvantage in the use of 3-MC is the large amount of oil and hydrocarbon required to induce mammary cancer by a single feeding. Other aromatics are far more effective than 3-MC. The most potent mammary carcinogens for rat are 7,12-DMBA and 7,8,12-TMBA but these compounds cause selective destruction of the adrenal cortex and sometimes completely destroy the bone marrow.

7,12-Dimethylbenz[a]*anthracene by Gastric Instillation.* A single tube-feeding (method 6.1) of 7,12-DMBA is highly effective in producing mammary cancer under stipulated conditions. A feeding of a solution of 7,12-DMBA in vegetable oil at various dose levels was given on a solitary occasion to groups of female S-D rats, age 50 days, and the induction of mammary cancer and the number of active centers were observed. In a few rats 7,12-DMBA (1 mg) induced mammary cancer, and there was a steady rise in the incidence of cancers with increased dosage until the optimal quantity was reached (fig. 6.2). The optimal dose of 7,12-DMBA, dissolved in sesame oil 2 ml, was 20 mg (130 mg/kg), for: *i*, every rat survived; *ii*, mammary cancer developed in each member of a series of 38 rats; *iii*, the

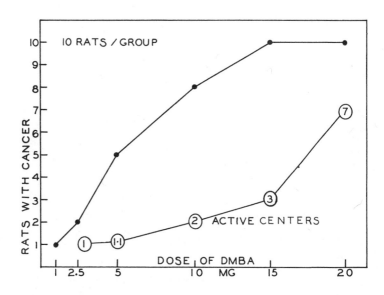

Fig. 6.2. Incidence of mammary cancer in groups of 10 S-D rats age 50 days fed 7, 12-DMBA once only. The average number of active centers in each group is given.

first cancer was palpable on day 24 and all rats had visible cancers of the breast within 2 months; and *iv*, the number of active centers in individual rats varied from 3 to 21 (the average was 7). A single meal of 15 mg of 7,12-DMBA dissolved in 2 ml of sesame oil elicited cancers of the breast in every rat but there were fewer active centers (fig. 6.2).

Method 6.1: Induction of Mammary Cancer by a Single Feeding of 7,12-DMBA

7,12-DMBA, mp 122–123°C (Eastman Kodak Co., Rochester, (N.Y.), was purified by Florisil chromatography and recrystallized from acetone-ethyl alcohol. A solution of refined 7,12-DMBA, 1% wt/vol, in sesame oil was prepared by heating the mixture for 30 min at 100°C. The solution was protected from light. Gastric tubes made from soft rubber catheters (size No. 8 Fr) had the following dimensions: length 6 cm; outside diameter 2.7 mm. Female rats of S-D strain, age 50 days, were anesthetized lightly with ether and tube fed with a single feeding of 2 ml of the solution containing 20 mg of 7,12-DMBA (∼ 130 mg/kg).

Tumors are induced selectively (table 6.3) by 7,12-DMBA. These include mammary carcinoma, mammary fibroadenoma, leukemia, and squamous carcinoma of sebaceous glands (Zymbal 1933) adjacent to the external auditory canal. The first three classes occur in untreated S-D rats (table 6.3), whereas ear duct tumors of spontaneous origin have never been observed in our laboratory.

Table 6.3   Incidence of Neoplasms in Female Albino Rats Fed 7,12-DMBA and Their Untreated Controls

Tumors	Number	Percent	Time of detection (days) Range	Time of detection (days) Mean
a. 164 Control Rats Received no 7,12-DMBA				
Mammary cancer	2	1.2	53–101	—
Fibroadenoma	10	6.1	137–208	167 ± 53
Lymphosarcoma	1	0.6	120	—
Ear duct cancer	0	—	—	—
b. 38 Rats Fed 7,12-DMBA, 20 mg, at age 50 days				
Mammary cancer	38	100	24– 61	39 ± 6
Fibroadenoma	34	89	147–209	194 ± 38
Leukemia	1	2.5	147	—
Ear duct cancer	2	5	146–246	—

NOTE: A single feeding of 7,12-DMBA was given by gastric tube to group *b*. Means with standard deviation ± are given.

Gruenstein et al. 1966 compared the effectiveness of the intragastric instillation of 3-MC (given by repeated feedings) with a solitary meal of 7,12-DMBA vis-à-vis the production of mammary cancer; two strains of albino rats were studied. It was found that S-D rats are more susceptible than Wistar rats are and that 7,12-DMBA is more active as a mammary carcinogen than 3-MC is (table 6.2).

The feces are intensely fluorescent following the administration of hydrocarbons by gastric instillation. Whereas the administration of 7,12-DMBA by tube feeding is highly efficient as a method to induce mammary cancer in young female S-D rats, the compound need not traverse the entire gastrointestinal tract for sufficient absorption of the carcinogen to cause mammary cancer. The injection of 7,12-DMBA (20 mg) into the lumen of the colon caused the development of mammary cancer in many rats (Huggins, Morii, and Grand 1961). But 7,12-DMBA need not traverse any part of the intestine to elicit cancer. A single intravenous injection of 7,12-DMBA prepared as a fine emulsion produced mammary cancer (Huggins, Grand, and Brillantes 1961) in every rat under the stipulated conditions.

Carcinogenic Emulsions for Intravenous Injection

The production of mammary adenocarcinoma in young female albino rats by a single pulse-injection (method 6.2) of homogenized aromatic hydrocarbons is a useful method in research on cancer of the breast. The technique is simple and the results are spectacular.

Method 6.2: Induction of Mammary Cancer in Albino Rat by Pulse-Injections of Emulsions of 7,12-DMBA or 7,8,12-TMBA

The aromatic hydrocarbon, 7,12-DMBA, mp 122–123°C, was refined (method 6.1). The carcinogen, 7,8,12-TMBA, mp 127–128°C, was synthesized (Bachmann and Chemerda 1938). Lipid emulsions containing a single hydrocarbon were prepared by the method of Schurr 1969 (appendix 2); 1 gm of the emulsion contained 150 mg of cottonseed oil, 12 mg of lecithin and 5 mg of the hydrocarbon.

The recipients were female S-D rats, age 25–65 days. The animal was restrained in a heavy cotton glove, permitting the tail to stick outside. The tail was immersed in warm water (48°C) for 1–2 min. A syringe with hypodermic needle (No. 26–29 gauge) was used to inject the emulsion in a caudal vein. Under stated conditions mammary cancer is elicited in high yield ($\sim$ 100%) by a single intravenous injection of 7,12-DMBA, 35 mg/kg, or of 7,8,12-TMBA, 35 mg/kg.

Mammary cancers arise regularly and rapidly after a solitary intravenous injection of the strong carcinogenic emulsions.

Proposition 3: Induction of Mammary Cancer

Under stated conditions, every female rat of Sprague-Dawley strain given one intravenous injection of 7,12-dimethylbenz[a]-anthracene, 35 mg/kg, or 7,8,12-trimethylbenz[a]anthracene, 35 mg/kg, at age 50 days will develop mammary adenocarcinoma or leukemia.

There are two factors that make the concentrated carcinogenic emulsions possible: *i*, the exceptional lipophilic solubility of 7,12-DMBA and 7,8-12-TMBA, and *ii*, the outstanding carcinogenicity of these two compounds, which elicit cancer of the breast quickly after a small dose has been given.

The solubility (wt/vol) of carcinogenic hydrocarbons in vegetable oil at 25°C was estimated: 3-MC $\sim$ 2%; 3'Me-DAB $\sim$ 2%; benzo[a]pyrene $\sim$ 5%; 7,12-DMBA $\sim$ 5%; 7,8,12-TMBA $\sim$ 10%. Of these aromatics 3'Me-DAB does not cause mammary cancer; it is a hepatic carcinogen which elicits tumors of the liver when incorporated in the ration. The remaining aromatics produce mammary cancer preferentially rather than neoplasms of the liver, which arise rarely. Emulsions of each aromatic were prepared by the method of Schurr 1969 (appendix 2). In eliciting cancer of the breast, emulsions of 7,12-

DMBA and 7,8,12-TMBA are more effective than all other chemical compounds by ten times.

In an emulsion each fat droplet is a nonaqueous solution which contains all of the compounds that have preferential solubility in lipids. The concentrated cancer-producing emulsions of Schurr 1969 are sterile and stable and have retained full cancer-producing potency for more than 10 years at 4°C. Intravenous injections of emulsions of carcinogens have many advantages, including: sudden introduction of a known amount of compound in the blood at a precise instant of time, extreme simplicity (method 6.2), convenience, saving of rare and costly materials, protection of personnel from potentially hazardous substances, and absence of gastrointestinal irritation.

Geyer et al. 1951 were the first to prepare lipid emulsions of 7,12-DMBA; these were injected intravenously in rats under ether anesthesia in sets of multiple injections. The Geyer emulsions contained $\sim 0.04\%$ of 7,12-DMBA. Administration of ca. 5 mg of 7,12-DMBA/100 gm body weight produced a tumor incidence of ca. 90% in 19 weeks (Geyer et al. 1953); most of the tumors were mammary adenocarcinoma or squamous carcinoma of sebaceous glands adjacent to the ear. No tumors were elicited by emulsions of 3-MC or benzo[a]pyrene.

In our laboratory emulsions containing 3'Me-DAB (0.5% wt/vol) were prepared by Schurr's method. Each of 20 L-E rats, males and females, received 10 intravenous injections of the emulsions at intervals of 3 days; the total dose of compound for each rat was 150 mg. No tumors were found during observation for 4 months.

Special 15% fat emulsions with 7,12-DMBA, 5 mg/gm, were prepared by the method of Schurr 1969 (appendix 2). The emulsions (p. 180) were made in a high-pressure homogenizing system; 97% of the oil was in emulsion droplets ≤ 1 μm in diameter, whereas particles larger than 5 μm were rarely observed. These emulsions are stable and effective for 10+ years.

7,12-DMBA Injected in Newborn Rat. The toxicity of 7,12-DMBA in newborn rats was determined. On the day of their birth, S-D rats weighing $\sim$ 6 g were injected intraperitoneally with an emulsion of 7,12-DMBA, 0.25% w/v, and the dose of hydrocarbon causing the death of half of the animals was determined; the LD_{50} was 50 mg/kg (0.3 mg per rat).

Fifteen newborn female S-D rats were given a single intraperitoneal injection of 0.05 cc of a lipid emulsion containing 7,12-DMBA, 0.25 mg; the dose was 40 mg/kg. Mammary carcinoma arose in 8 rats (53%); it was detected at age 56–146 days. Intraperitoneal tumors did not occur (Huggins and Fuku-nishi 1963*b*). The histology of the mammary glands of new-born rats is shown in figure 6.3*A, B.*

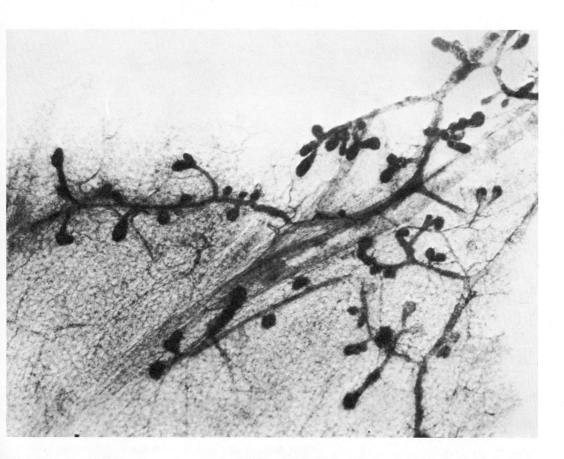

Fig. 6.3*A.* Histology of mammary glands of newborn rat. Whole mount of mammary gland of S-D rat, on birthday, in which the sites of alkaline phosphatase have been demonstrated. x90.

7,12-DMBA Injected in Prepubertal Female Rat. Twenty-five immature S-D female rats, age 25 days, were given a single intravenous injection of 0.5 cc of a lipid emulsion containing 7,12-DMBA (2.5 mg); the dose was ~ 38 mg/kg. The onset of puberty, defined by the day of the first estrus, was determined in this series; puberty occurred at age 30–39 days. Mammary cancers, elicited in every rat, were found in 50.8 ± 22 days (fig. 6.4); no other neoplasms were detected in the observation period of 4 months. The first mammary cancer was detected on day 31. At necropsy the adrenals were not calcified.

7,12-DMBA Injected in Young Adult Female Rat. Twenty-five S-D female rats, age 50 days, were given a single intra-

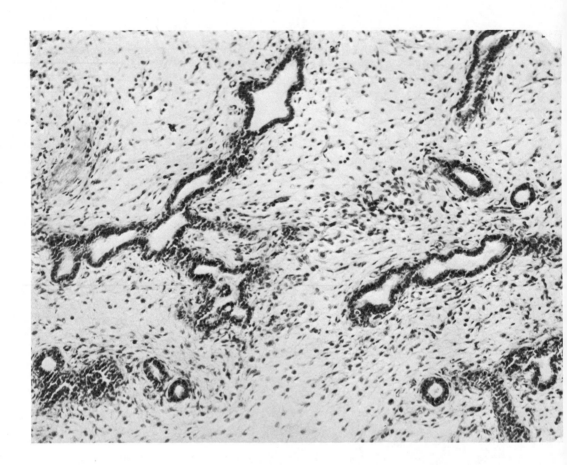

Fig. 6.3B. Histology of mammary glands of newborn rat. Histological section of mammary gland of S-D rat, on birthday. H. & E., x180.

venous injection of 1.0 cc of a lipid emulsion containing 7,12-DMBA (5 mg); the dose was ~ 38 mg/kg. All of the animals had had estrus cycles before the pulse-injection of the mammary carcinogen. Mammary cancer, elicited in every rat, was found in 41.9 ± 10 days (fig. 6.4). The number of active centers was 2.9. At necropsy sandlike calcification was found in the adrenals of every rat.

In eliciting mammary cancer in S-D female rats by a single dose of 7,12-DMBA given at age 50 days, the results of a solitary feeding or intravenous injection do not differ significantly (fig. 6.5).

Mammary cancers were induced in 20 female S-D rats, age 50 days, by a single intravenous injection of a lipid emulsion of 7,8,12-TMBA, 35 mg/kg. The mammary cancers were detected in 22–66 days, mean 41.1 ± 15 days. The number of active centers was 3.6.

Mammary Cancer in Ovariex Rat

Normal function of the ovaries greatly favors the presence of mammary cancer, both in its genesis and growth, in S-D female rat given an effective dose of 7,12-DMBA during the extremely sensitive first bimester of life. Cancer of the breast seldom arises in rats deprived of the ovaries unless the carcinogen is given soon after ovariectomy. In the experiments now to be described, mammary cancer was produced in a considerable proportion of ovariex rats treated with a cancer-producing dose of 7,12-DMBA under special conditions. In brief, we found a carry-over of susceptibility to the development of mammary cancer that persisted for 7–10 days after ovariectomy; the vulnerability to the production of cancer by 7,12-DMBA disappeared in the atrophic mammary tubules 3–4 weeks following removal of the ovaries (Sydnor and Cockrell 1963).

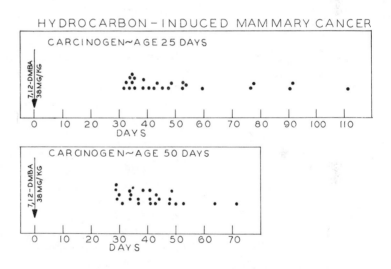

Fig. 6.4. Day of detection (●) of palpable mammary cancer in two groups of female S-D rats that received a single intravenous injection of 7,12-DMBA, 38 mg/kg, at age 25 or 50 days. The incidence of cancer of the breast in each group was 25 of 25 rats.

At age 23 days, the ovaries of 38 weanling S-D rats were removed; at age 25 days each rat received an intravenous injection of 2.5 mg of 7,12-DMBA (35 mg/kg) and the animals were observed for 200 days thereafter. The number of rats with malignant tumors (fig. 6.6) was 12 with mammary cancer, 14 of the ear duct, 7 of the kidney, and 3 of the skin. Some of the rats had multiple tumors; all of the neoplasms were carcinomas; 8 rats were tumor-free at day 200.

In another experiment, 10 S-D rats were subjected to ovariectomy at age 43 days, whereas 10 controls were not operated upon; at age 50 days, members of each group received an intravenous injection of 7,12-DMBA (40 mg/kg). The incidence

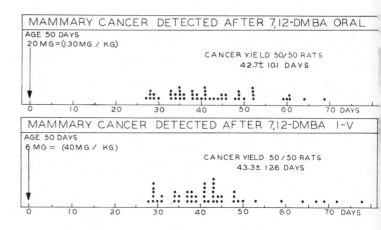

Fig. 6.5. In eliciting mammary cancer in S-D female rats by a single dose of 7,12-DMBA, given at age 50 days, the results of feeding and intravenous injection do not differ significantly.

of mammary cancer (with the time of appearance of the tumors) in the two groups was 10 out of 10 control rats (66.3 ± 16 days) and 9 out of 10 ovariex rats (78.4 ± 8 days).

In yet another experiment, 10 S-D rats were subjected to ovariectomy at age 43 days, whereas 10 control sisters were not operated upon. After 3 weeks, that is at age 64 days, members of both groups received an intravenous injection of 7,12-DMBA (40 mg/kg). The incidence of mammary cancer (with the time of appearance of the tumors) was 10 out of 10 control rats (52.2 ± 18 days) and 1 of 10 ovariex rats (175 days).

In ovariex rats vulnerability to carcinogen-induced mammary cancer was restored, when it had been lost, with small doses of estrogen. It was found that the injection of small doses of estradiol (0.5 μg/day) initiated mitosis and restored the susceptibility of the inactive mammary gland of ovariex rats so that mammary cancer ensued in every recipient exposed to a carcinogenic feeding of 7,12-DMBA (130 mg/kg).

Mammary Cancer in Hypox Rat

A rat deprived of the pituitary will survive for a prolonged period on a high protein diet. In the experiments of Huggins, Grand, and Brillantes 1959, 13 hypox rats lived more than 10 months after multiple feedings of 3-MC, 10 mg, which were given by gastric tube once each week for 7 weeks; no neoplasms of any sort were observed in any rat, whereas in a group of 9 intact control rats treated similarly with 3-MC mammary cancer developed in every one.

Young 1961 described the induction of mammary carcinoma in hypox rats that were treated by feeding 3-MC together with the injection of steroids and bovine growth hormone (BGH).

The pituitary of female S-D rats was removed at age 50 days. Hormone treatments were begun 13 days after hypophysectomy according to the following scheme: *i*, estradiol, 1 μg *plus* progesterone, 4 mg, subcutaneously daily for 6 days each week; *ii*, 3-MC, 10 mg intragastrically once each week; *iii*, BGH, 0.5 mg, daily. Mammary adenocarcinoma developed in 5 of 9 hypox rats treated in this way.

Molecular Characteristics of Mammary Carcinogens

Many substances (table 6.4) with divergent molecular structures possess in common the property of inducing mammary cancer selectively and rapidly after a single oral or intravenous dose. The effect appears to be related to participation in a molecular complex by an aromatic hydrocarbon possessing a prerequisite three-dimensional geometric configuration (Huggins and Yang 1962).

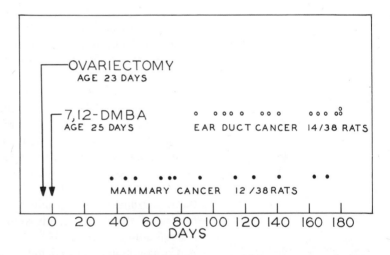

Fig. 6.6 Detection of ear duct and mammary cancers in prepubertal S-D rats subjected to removal of ovaries at age 23 days followed by intravenous injection of 7,12-DMBA, 35 mg/kg, at age 25 days.

Benz[*a*]anthracene (I in table 6.4) did not evoke mammary cancer; the addition of one methyl group in either *meso* position to form 12-methyl- (II) or 7-methylbenz[*a*]anthracene (III) resulted in a weak mammary carcinogen. The addition of 2 methyl groups to benz[*a*]anthracene to form 7,12-DMBA (IV) resulted in an extremely powerful carcinogen; an additional methyl group to form 7,8,12-trimethylbenz[*a*]anthracene profoundly modified toxicity of the compound—a decrease in rat and an increase in mouse (p. 160). The presence of methyl groups endowed the molecule benz[*a*]anthracene, otherwise inactive, with the ability to induce cancer. The addition of a salient alicyclic ring had an effect similar to that of methyl

Table 6.4   Induction of Mammary Cancer by a Single Feeding of Aromatic Hydrocarbons to S-D Female Rats Age 50 Days

Number	Compound	Dose (mg)	Rats (no.)	Mammary cancer (no.)	Percent
I	Benz[a]anthracene	200	18	0	0
II	12-Methylbenz[a]anthracene	100	12	2	17
III	7-Methylbenz[a]anthracene	100	13	4	31
IV	7,12-Dimethylbenz[a]anthracene	20	700	700	100
V	3-Methylcholanthrene	100	100	100	100
VI	Benzo[a]pyrene	100	9	8	89
VII	Phenanthrene	200	10	0	0
VIII	2-Aminophenanthrene	70	10	10	100
IX	2,4,7-Trinitro-9-fluorenone	100	20	7	35
X	4-Nitroquinoline-N-oxide	20	10	2	20

groups—for example, the addition of a cyclopenteno ring across the 7 and 8 positions of benz[a]anthracene forms the strongly carcinogenic cholanthrene; 3-methylcholanthrene (V) in big doses is a mammary carcinogen. Alternatively, the extension of an extra aromatic ring converts benz[a]anthracene to benzo[a]-pyrene (VI), a highly carcinogenic compound.

Phenanthrene (VII) is not carcinogenic but 2-aminophenanthrene (VIII) is a strong carcinogen. In common with other aromatic amines, a big dose of 2-aminophenanthrene oxidizes hemoglobin and produces methemoglobinemia. The aromatic amines induced sleep; hence 2-aminophenanthrene is an anesthetic carcinogen. The smallest mammary carcinogens possess two rings; structures of this kind are 4-aminodiphenyl and 4-nitroquinoline-N-oxide (X).

The compounds I–VIII have the phenanthrene structure but an ethylene bridge between aromatic rings is adequate; 4-dimethylaminostilbene synthesized by Haddow et al. 1948 is a moderately effective mammary carcinogen (Huggins 1962), whereas stilbene did not produce cancer.

All of the special carcinogens are flat molecules with conjugated double-bond systems and possess substituent groups of a special sort or (what is equivalent) an additional ring at a salient position in the molecule.

We see that the parent molecular species (benz[a]anthracene, phenanthrene, stilbene, fluorene) are devoid of carcinogenic activity; the potency of aromatic hydrocarbons in inciting cancer depends on the contribution of substituents or an additional ring at a special site. Substituents with effective potency in converting an otherwise inactive molecule to a powerful carcinogen are methyl groups and also amino groups and their derivatives dimethylamino and acetylamino. The addition of an extra aromatic ring to benz[*a*]anthracene creates a compound, benzo[*a*]pyrene, which is nearly as effective as 7,12-DMBA. The common property of -CH$_3$, -NH$_2$, and the salient aromatic rings is their ability to donate electrons to appropriate acceptors as π-donors or N-donors. Szent-Györgyi, Isenberg, and Baird 1960 observed that the carcinogenicity of aromatic hydrocarbons is correlated with their ability to form charge transfer complexes with local acceptors such as I:I. Szent-Györgyi, Isenberg, and Baird 1960 state, "Carcinogenicity of these substances is connected with their ability to form strong charge transfer complexes with local acceptors and give off an electron."

A common property of the cancer-producing aromatics is that they readily engage in the formation of colored molecular complexes with electron acceptors such as iodine, nitroaromatics, cyanoaromatics, and quinones. Such complexes usually occur between one molecule of the aromatic hydrocarbon and one molecule of the acceptor and are of the so-called donor-acceptor type. These complexes absorb light (and hence exhibit unstructured absorption bands) at longer wavelengths than either aromatic donor or electron acceptor. The new color, resulting from formation of the complex, is caused by the fact that, when light is absorbed a π-electron (one of the loosely bound electrons involved in formation of double bonds) from the donor is excited into an unfilled molecular orbital of the acceptor. In other words, excitation of the complex leads to a transfer of an electron from aromatic carcinogen to the acceptor. But even in the ground state of the complex (i.e., in the absence of exciting electromagnetic radiation) there is some degree of intermolecular donor-acceptor interaction (Foster 1969).

The carcinogenic compounds II–VI, and VIII are powerful electron donors that form strong donor-acceptor complexes with electron acceptors, for example, trinitrofluorenone and trinitrobenzene. It was surprising to learn that the strong electron acceptors 2,4,7-trinitro-9-fluorenone (IX) and 4-nitroquinoline-N-oxide (X) are also rather powerful mammary carcinogens under conditions indicated in table 6.4. It would appear that aromatics that are either strong electron donors or acceptors can induce cancer.

But electronic factors per se are not enough to cause cancer; steric factors also are involved. Yang et al. 1961 showed that there is a direct increase in carcinogenicity as aromatic hydro-carbons become sterically similar to steroid hormones.

There is a remarkable similarity in geometric two-dimensional pattern (but not in molecular thickness) between carcinogenic polynuclear aromatic hydrocarbons, growth-promoting steroids, and the base pairs of nucleic acids. This was easily demon-strated. A molecular model was made of guanine-cytosine and a frame was constructed to surround it (Huggins and Yang 1962). In this frame similar atomic models of progesterone, testosterone, and estradiol-17β fit neatly. Similarly all mammary carcinogens (table 6.4) can be inserted in this frame. The poly-nuclear aromatic carcinogens have an identical thickness (3.6 Å) to the base pairs. The steroids are not carcinogenic vis-à-vis the mammary glands of our colony of S-D females, and it would appear that they are excluded from mammary carcinogenicity because steroids are not planar; the thickness of the steroid molecules (ca. 5–6 Å) far exceeds that of base pairs and would preclude intercalation in the ladderlike double-stranded struc-ture of DNA.

The hypothesis of Huggins and Yang 1962 states that there are three molecular factors of critical significance determining mamary carcinogenicity in polynuclear aromatic hydrocarbons and aromatic amines: *i*, the electron transfer factor, *ii*, the geo-metric factor (the configuration must resemble that of steroids and of the purine-pyrimidine pairs of DNA), and *iii*, molecular thickness which must not exceed the thickness of the base pairs. In brief, the mammary carcinogens must resemble the base pairs of nucleic acids in three-dimensional geometric configura-tion and be able to participate in donor-acceptor complexes.

Biological Characteristics of Mammary Carcinoma

The superficial position of the mammary glands permits ready detection of mammary cancer by palpation. The end point is sharp; the cancers are discrete and shotlike. A tumor weighing 8–10 mg can be detected easily and with high accuracy, but subsequent growth of the mass and its histological verification are desirable to confirm the diagnosis. The cancers arise any-where in the mammary tissue, which is distributed on rat's ven-tral surface from neck to perineum; there is no favored site of predilection. In their incipient stage all of the mammary cancers are firm in consistency; some infiltrate the overlying skin; others are nodules, pinhead to split pea in size, in the subcutaneous fat. After a single dose of carcinogen mammary cancers have been found by histological examination in 11 days and by palpa-tion in 20 days. The early mammary cancers have always been apparent in clusters of multiple adjacent tumors (fig. 6.7) rather than individual solitary neoplastic masses. The mammary cancers rarely metastasize; they kill by attaining gigantic size and by invading adjacent tissues with consequent hemorrhage, necrosis, and ulceration. Metastases can be produced readily; in the experiments of Dao 1964 autologous mammary cancer cells, which were injected in the rat's portal vein, produced multiple colonies of mammary carcinoma in the liver.

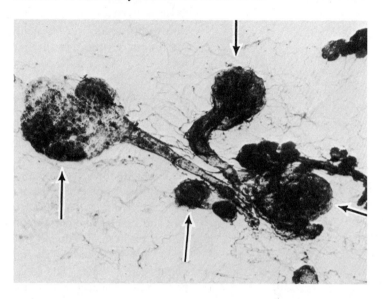

Fig. 6.7. Whole mount of mammary glands of S-D female rat; alkaline phosphatase preparation. Arrows point to a cluster of early mammary cancers induced by repeated feedings of 3-MC. Normal mammary acini are on the right.

The carcinomas evoked by irradiation or carcinogenic hydrocarbons in intact rats have a considerable similarity of cytologic pattern. The tumors consist of acini lined with many layers of epithelial cells arranged to form glandlike structures with papillary projections; the lumina of these malignant glands were filled with eosinophilic mucoprotein, which stained deeply with mucicarmine and the PAS reagents. The alkaline phosphatase reaction (fig. 6.7) served to identify the myoepithelial cells, which were present in great numbers and were irregularly organized around and within the neoplastic glands.

The mammary carcinomas induced with aromatics in ovariex rats differed morphologically from the neoplasms elicited in intact rats. The chief difference was in the epithelial cells and in the secretion of the tumor acini in the spayed rats. Whereas in both intact and ovariex rats there occurred neoplastic glandlike structures lined with many layers of cells and surrounded by myoepithelial cells, the secretion in the lumina of the tumor acini of ovariex animals was devoid of alkaline phosphatase and mucoprotein (Huggins, Briziarelli, and Sutton 1959). In the mammary tumors of spayed rats, some of the acini were lined with a single row of flat cells while other glands consisted of many layers of epithelial cells.

Enzymes in Mammary Carcinoma

Warburg 1930 discovered that a high rate of aerobic glycolysis is a metabolic characteristic of all active malignant disease. Meister 1950 observed that the levels of lactic dehydrogenase in tumors of rodents are frequently higher than in the corresponding tissues of origin. Both effects obtain in mammary cancer in rat.

The mammary glands of virgin female rats consist of slender tubules embedded in much fat. This preponderance of lipocytes makes it difficult to study the metabolic characteristics of the mammary tubules in virgins; hence in our work biochemical characteristics of mammary cancers were compared with those of the hyperplastic mammary glands of pregnant or lactating rats. To eliminate the contribution of fat to the gross weight of tissue, which would influence enzyme values in the normal mammary glands, all values were calculated in terms of units/mg protein/min and this is denoted specific activity.

The respiration values (Rees and Huggins 1960) of mammary cancers are similar to those of normal lactating mammary glands ($Qo_2 \sim 12$). The respiration of slices of mammary cancer increased nearly twofold in the presence of 2,4-dinitrophenol because of the uncoupling of oxidation and oxidative phosphorylation. Hydrocarbon-induced mammary cancer had the high aerobic glycolysis that is distinctive of the metabolism of neoplasms. The rate of glycolysis decreased in the presence of oxygen (Pasteur effect).

The levels of lactic dehydrogenase (LDH), malic dehydrogenase (MDH), and alkaline phosphatase were determined (method 6.3) in mammary cancer and in the nonmalignant mammary hyperplasias (Huggins, Oka, and Fareed 1972). In the hyperplasias of pregnancy and lactation and in mammary cancer as well the levels of both LDH and MDH exceed by several orders of magnitude the values of other pyridine nucleotide-linked dehydrogenases (Rees and Huggins 1960).

Method 6.3:
Enzyme Assays

Tissues were excised rapidly, weighed on a torsion balance, and homogenized in an ice-cold solution of 0.15M NaCl containing 0.0003M $NaHCO_3$; 40–80 mg of tissue was disintegrated in

2 ml of the buffered saline in a Polytron homogenizer with three 10-second bursts. The homogenate was centrifuged at 11,000 $\times$ g in a refrigerated centrifuge; enzyme assays were performed on the supernatant.

Lactic Dehydrogenase (EC 1.1.1.27). The substrate for LDH was 0.003M sodium pyruvate dissolved in 0.0833M Tris buffer, pH 7.4, containing 0.0001M NADH.

Malic Dehydrogenase (EC 1.1.1.37). The substrate for MDH was 0.001M sodium oxalacetate dissolved in 0.0833M Tris buffer, pH 7.4, containing 0.0001M NADH.

Menadione Reductase (EC 1.6.99.2). The substrate for MR was 0.0001M menadione dissolved in 0.0833M Tris buffer, pH 7.4, containing 0.0001M NADH. Menadione dissolved in ethanol was added subsurface to the aqueous phase, which was stirred vigorously with a magnet.

Three ml of reaction mixture was placed in a silica cuvette of 1 cm light path and 0.02 ml of homogenate was added to start the reaction. The initial rate of oxidation of NADH at 25°C was measured for 1 min in a Beckman DU spectrophotometer; the optimal enzyme concentration yielded an absorbance change of 0.015–0.025 OD units/mg/min at 340 mμ.

One unit of LDH or MDH or MR is defined as that activity which oxidizes 1 μmole of NADH/min/g of tissue under the specified conditions.

The concentration of protein was determined by the method of Lowry et al. 1951. Specific activity is defined as units/mg protein/min.

LDH isozymes were separated by electrophoresis on a cellulose slide in a mixture (1:1) of 0.2M Tris buffer pH 8.3 and 0.075M sodium barbital pH 8.6. The relative migration and concentration of isozymes was measured in an electrophoresis densitometer. The isozymes are designated H_4(LDH$_1$), H_3M(LDH$_2$), H_2M$_2$(LDH$_3$), HM$_3$(LDH$_4$) and M$_4$(LDH$_5$).

Alkaline phosphatase was determined by the method of Huggins and Morii 1961. One unit of alkaline phosphatase liberates 1 μmole of p-nitrophenol/0.5 hr/g of tissue at 38°C.

The hyperplastic mammary glands in pregnancy (day 8 or 13) contained no milk; the level of MDH exceeded that of LDH (table 6.5); the ratio LDH/MDH was less than unity (Huggins, Oka, and Fareed 1972).

Table 6.5   Alkaline Phosphatase and Lactic and Malic Dehydrogenases in
Hyperlastic Mammary Glands and Mammary Cancer

	Alkaline Phosphatase	LDH	MDH	LDH/MDH*
Pregnancy, day 8				
Units/g	15.3 ± 5.0	13.6 ± 2.3	37.9 ± 15.6	0.36
Units/mg protein	0.52 ± 0.11	0.48 ± 0.12	1.32 ± 0.54	
Pregnancy, day 13				
Units/g	25.5 ± 10.4	16.4 ± 3.3	44.2 ± 11.2	0.37
Units/mg protein	0.92 ± 0.26	0.61 ± 0.12	1.66 ± 0.39	
Lactation, day 6				
Units/g	51.5 ± 13.9	67.7 ± 11.7	163.5 ± 15.1	0.41
Units/mg protein	0.58 ± 0.14	0.77 ± 0.14	1.87 ± 0.25	
Mammary cancer				
Units/g	14.3 ± 7.6	192.7 ± 36.8	137.8 ± 36.9	1.41
Units/mg protein	0.21 ± 0.11	2.12 ± 0.43	1.63 ± 0.52	

NOTE: The rats were females of L-E strain. There were 8 rats in each
group. Tumors were induced by pulse-doses of 7,8,12-TMBA. The results
are expressed in units/g of tissue, wet weight, and as specific activity.
Means with standard deviation ± are given.
*LDH/MDH is the ratio of LDH to MDH.

The hyperplastic mammary glands in lactation (postpartum
day 6) secreted milk copiously; as in pregnancy the level of
MDH exceeded that of LDH; the ratio LDH/MDH was less
than unity.

An important difference between the normal hyperplasia and
mammary cancer was the absolute and relative increase in concentration of LDH in carcinoma of the breast of the rat (Huggins, Oka, and Fareed 1972); always in mammary cancer (rat)
the ratio LDH/MDH was greater than unity (table 6.5).

In all normal states of proliferation of mammary gland the
pattern of isozymes in mammary gland was similar to that of
skeletal muscle; in mammary cancer the most striking finding
is an absolute increase in enzymes of skeletal muscle type with
no detection of H_4 or H_3M isozymes.

Rees and Huggins 1960 found that many mammary cancers
of rats that had been treated with large doses of estradiol secreted large quantities of milk with a vast accumulation of lipids
in the epithelial cells. The lipid concentration in some of the
tumors was 16%–35% (wt/wt) and the cancers floated in
water. Lactation in the mammary carcinomas of rat and dog (p.
55) was a newly recognized attribute of hormonal responsivity.

Estrogen Receptors in Experimental Mammary Cancer

King, Cowan, and Inman 1965 studied the uptake and intracellular localization of [³H]estradiol in liver and mammary adenocarcinoma of female S-D rats treated with 7,12-DMBA. The tumor is similar to other estrogen-responsive tissues in that the major estrogen is estradiol, which is mainly associated with cell nuclei. The tumor has the ability to retain the estrogen for more than 4 hr. Estrogen was not retained by the liver cells.

Jensen et al. 1972b found that those mammary cancers induced by 7,12-DMBA which are hormone-dependent resemble uterus and vagina in their affinity for estradiol; the hormone is incorporated without chemical transformation. The tumor is sensitive to Nafoxidine and other binding inhibitors; these depress the uptake of estradiol. Detailed study of the interaction of estradiol with the 7,12-DMBA-induced mammary cancers demonstrates that this proceeds by the two-step mechanism described by Jensen et al. 1968; an 8S receptor protein in the cytosol dissociable into 4S subunits serves as the precursor of the 5S estradiol-receptor complex extractable from the nucleus. A small fraction, ca. 10%–12%, of the induced carcinomas are nondependent, inasmuch as they do not regress after ovariectomy; the uptake of estradiol by these nonregressing tumors was present but considerably smaller than the dependent ones.

Boylan and Witliff 1975 found that hormone-dependent mammary cancers induced by 7,12-DMBA in the rat undergo interaction with [³H]estradiol. It was noteworthy that certain of the rat's mammary carcinomas which continued to grow after ovariectomy contained significant amounts of estradiol bound to cytoplasmic as well as nuclear components.

Genetic Constitution, Mammary Cancer, and Endocrine Status of Rat Strains

There is a profound difference between two strains (S-D and L-E) of rats in their susceptibility to mammary cancer, which is reflected in the incidence of spontaneous mammary cancer and in the development of cancer of the mammary gland after a massive but tolerable feeding or pulse-injection of 7,12-DMBA or 7,8,12-TMBA. In addition there are differences in the rate of body growth, the rate at which the strains reached sexual maturity, and the reaction to the toxicity of the aromatics.

S-D female rats have the following characteristics:

1. The incidence of spontaneous mammary cancer was 1.2%.
2. One pulse-dose of 7,8,12-TMBA, 35 mg/kg, elicited mammary cancer in every animal (100%) injected at age 50 days and the neoplasms were palpable at 42 ± 11 days.
3. Three biweekly pulse-injections of 7,8,12-TMBA, 35

mg/kg, caused the death of all of the rats within 31 days.

4. The rats were highly susceptible to pneumonitis.

5. The females exhibited early rapid growth and early sexual maturity.

L-E female rats have the following characteristics:

1. The incidence of spontaneous mammary cancer was 0.

2. One pulse-dose of 7,8,12-TMBA, 35 mg/kg, elicited mammary cancer in 0–8%.

3. Multiple pulse-injections of 7,8,12-TMBA, 35 mg/kg, at biweekly intervals resulted in little mortality and elicited mammary cancer and leukemia in high yields.

4. The rats were resistant to pneumonitis and other intercurrent infections.

5. The females exhibited slower increment of body mass (fig. 6.8) and later sexual maturity than S-D females did.

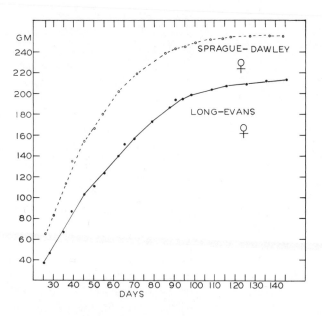

Fig. 6.8. Curves of body weight of normal females of L-E and S-D strains.

The relation of race to the incidence of mammary cancer was investigated in S-D and L-E strains (Sydnor et al. 1962); the animals were heterozygous since the strains were bred at random inter se, not by brother $\times$ sister mating. The females had 1–3 estrus cycles. All rats were given a single feeding of 7,12-DMBA (130 mg/kg) at age 50–65 days and observed 6 months thereafter. Three genetic sets were investigated, purebred strains, F_1 hybrids, and the first backcross.

Purebred strains. All purebred S-D females (100%) given a single feeding of 7,12-DMBA (20 mg) developed mammary cancer (table 6.6). The cancers were detected in 25–74 days and they grew rapidly; the neoplasms required excision at intervals of 2–3 weeks because of considerable size and usually removal of 3–10 cancers per rat was needed at each seance.

Table 6.6   Mammary Cancer in S-D and L-E Strains and in Hybrids Thereof

Strain	Number of rats	Mammary Cancer	
		Number	Percent
S-D♀ x S-D♂	38	38	100
L-E♀ x L-E♂	25	4	16
S-D♀ x L-E♂, F_1	29	21	72
L-E♀ x S-D♂, F_1	26	20	77

NOTE: All rats received a single 20 mg feeding of 7,12-DMBA at age 50–65 days.

Under similar conditions few purebred L-E females (16%) developed mammary cancers; these were observed in 42–180 days and none required excision for lifesaving purposes.

F_1 hybrids. Mammary cancer developed in a considerable and nearly equal proportion in F_1 hybrids of reciprocal cross of S-D and L-E strains given a single feeding of 7,12-DMBA (130 mg/kg). The incidence of mammary cancer (table 6.6) was: S-D ♀ × L-E ♂, 72%; L-E ♀ × S-D ♂, 77%.

First backcross. Female F_1 hybrids were backcrossed with males of the original purebred S-D and L-E strains; the offspring were given a single feeding of 7,12-DMBA (20 mg) on the day of the first estrus. The preponderant genetic strain, whether S-D or L-E, exerted a profound influence on the incidence of mammary cancer. The incidence of mammary cancers in virgins of the first backcross was:

(S-D ♀ × L-E ♂) ♀ × S-D ♂ = 100%
(L-E ♀ × S-D ♂) ♀ × S-D ♂ = 89%
(S-D ♀ × L-E ♂) ♀ × L-E ♂ = 40%
(L-E ♀ × S-D ♂) ♀ × L-E ♂ = 28%

When most of the genetic material was derived from S-D strain, all or nearly all of the animals developed mammary cancer, whereas in the hybrids of predominantly L-E stock the incidence of mammary cancer was significantly lower. The susceptibility factor in mammary cancer is inherited as a dominant trait.

Growth Rate and   Compared with companions of S-D strain, L-E females had
Sexual Maturity   smaller initial body mass at age 25 days and slower rate of
                             growth thereafter (fig. 6.8). The vaginal plate opened later and
                             first estrus in L-E rats was significantly delayed (table 6.7).

Table 6.7   Onset of Puberty in Rats of L-E and S-D Strains

	Day of Vaginal Opening		Day of First Estrus	
Strain	Range	Mean	Range	Mean
L-E	33–63	44.3 ± 9	33–63	$50 \ \pm 6.5$
S-D	30–39	32.9 ± 3	30–39	34.5 ± 2.8

NOTE: There were 20 rats in each group. Means with standard deviation
± are given.

Apropos of experimental mammary cancer in mice, Bittner
1958*a* and *b* described two inherited hormonal patterns. Bittner
(1958*b*) stated: "One of these plays a role in the induction of
mammary tumors in virgin females, while another may inhibit
their development in breeding females of susceptible stocks with
the (mammary tumor) agent."

Sydnor et al. 1962 demonstrated that the ovary of L-E and
S-D rats responds similarly to gonadotrophin so that it may be
inferred that the considerable sexual and growth difference of
the females is related to a heritable difference in pituitary function in L-E and S-D strains.

Racial origin of the rat is significant in relation to mammary
cancer induced by a single dose of powerful carcinogenic aromatic hydrocarbon but resistance to mammary cancer vanishes
when multiple doses of the polycyclic compounds are given. In
the L-E strain a single intravenous injection of 5 mg of 7,12-
DMBA induced mammary cancer in 9% of the recipients; when
sisters were given a similar dose on 4 occasions the incidence
of cancer of the breast was 94% (Sydnor et al. 1962) and
many of the animals developed leukemia.

Item: Genus Homo. In 1956–57 the incidence of mammary
cancer in white women in the United States was 27.08/100,000;
the comparable incidence in Oriental women in Japan was 3.26
(Segi 1960).

7 Acceleration and Extinction of Mammary Cancer

Under stated conditions a solitary feeding (p. 73) or intravenous injection of 7,12-DMBA induces mammary carcinoma in young female albino rats selectively, rapidly, and in nearly every animal. The growth rate of the mammary cancer and indeed its very existence are controllable for a shorter or longer time, often lifelong, by methods of endocrinology. The techniques are versatile; the growth of the tumor can be accelerated or the cancer can be exterminated. To a large extent mammary carcinoma in rat, its presence and development, are under the control of the investigator.

The attribute whereby the acceleration of growth or the destruction of cancer cells is brought about by altering the endocrine status is designated hormone-responsiveness; it is a quality that resides in the cancer cell. The survival, rate of growth, and development of hormone-responsive cells are determined by the hormonal milieu interne of the host.

Proposition 4: Endocrine Extinction of Cancer

Hormone-responsive cancer cells can be destroyed by hormone deprivation or by hormone surplus—too little or too much, the methods are poles apart.

Proposition 5: Duration of Endocrine Responsiveness

Mammary cancers are hormone-responsive for at least 28 days following a solitary cancer-producing dose of 7,12-dimethylbenz[a]anthracene given to female rats of Sprague-Dawley strain at age 50 days.

Acceleration of the rate of growth of mammary cancers occurs during pregnancy and pseudopregnancy (Dao and Sunderland 1959) and following the administration of progesterone and related progestational agents (Huggins, Grand, and Brillantes 1959).

Extinction of hormone-responsive mammary cancer is brought about by hypophysectomy or, less frequently, by ovariectomy.

Extinction also occurs during lactation (Bielschowsky 1947) and following the administration of large amounts of dihydro-testosterone, estrogens, or equine gonadotrophin ' (Huggins, Grand, and Brillantes 1959). Procedures that produce florid estrus destroy mammary cancers. A combination of big doses of estradiol *plus* progesterone extinguishes without producing lactation (Huggins, Grand, and Brillantes 1959).

Hypophysectomy and Ovariectomy

Many of the induced mammary carcinomas of the rat undergo profound regression following the removal of the pituitary or the ovaries. The majority of these neoplasms vanish when endocrine ablation of these sorts is carried out soon after the tumor has been detected. In comparison with ovariectomy, removal of the pituitary is a more effective method to destroy hormone-responsive mammary cancer. The pituitary mammogenic hormones have high significance in the growth of hormone-responsive cancers of the breast.

In most of the strains of mice spontaneous mammary cancers that have reached palpable size do not regress following ovariectomy or hypophysectomy. The mouse tumors are seldom hormone-responsive in their later stages.

The involution of mammary cancer following ovariectomy or hypophysectomy is not due to necrosis but results from atrophy of the cancerous epithelial cells; a characteristic histologic appearance (p. 91) ensues.

At age 32 days (day 0), just before the onset of estrus, 69 female S-D rats received an intravenous injection of 7,12-DMBA, 36 mg/kg. In this series the first estrus occurred at age 36–50 days, mean 41.2 ± 5 days. On day 20, mammary cancer (fig. 7.1) was demonstrated by biopsy of an inguinal mammary gland of one of the rats.

On day 25 the first mammary cancer was detected by palpation. On day 32, the rats were separated into 3 groups, which were subjected to hypophysectomy, ovariectomy, or no operation. On day 136 the incidence (fig. 7.2) of mammary cancer was 100% of unoperated controls, 35% of ovariex, and 4% of hypox.

In the study of Kim and Furth 1960, 72% of carcinogen-induced mammary cancers were inhibited by ovariectomy and 86% by hypophysectomy. Most of the inhibited tumors remained minute in size; a few resumed growth and a moderate number (∼ 37% in the hypox series) could not be identified at necropsy. In hypox rats grafts of functional mammotrophic pituitary tumors (secreting somatotrophin and prolactin) caused

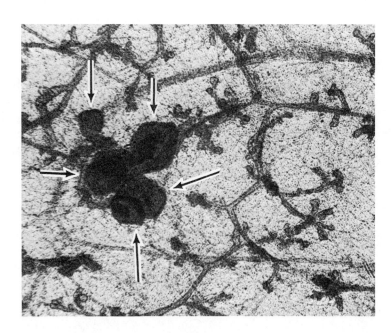

Fig. 7.1. Whole mount of mammary glands of S-D female rat, age 52 days, 20 days after intravenous injection of 7,12-DMBA, 36 mg/kg. The arrows point to a cluster of mammary cancers; most of the mammary acini are normal noncancerous glands.

not only resumption of progressive tumor growth of the inhibited neoplasms but the appearance of new mammary cancers.

Huggins, Briziarelli, and Sutton 1959 removed the ovaries or the pituitary from rats bearing large mammary cancers produced by feeding 3-MC. Following hypophysectomy, all of the tumors in a series of 9 rats underwent a profound decrease in size (fig. 7.3). At necropsy, in 2 rats small masses of mammary cancer (ca. 5 × 5 mm) were found 50 days following hypophysectomy, whereas in 7 rats no tumors were detected.

Ovariectomy was performed on 8 rats bearing carcinogen-induced cancer of the breast. In 7 rats the tumor underwent a considerable decrease in its size, whereas in one animal the tumor continued to grow despite deprival of the ovaries. There was a similar divergent effect of growth of mammary cancers in rats injected daily with dihydrotestosterone, 1 mg or 2 mg. This steroid was administered to 17 intact tumor-bearing animals; a considerable regression of mass of the mammary cancer occurred in 14 animals, whereas the tumor size continued to increase in 3 rats.

The mammary cancers that diminished in size after the endocrine modifications (hypophysectomy, ovariectomy, or administration of dihydrotestosterone) exhibited thereafter a characteristic cytologic appearance of atrophy of epithelial cells which was similar in all groups. The tumor acini were still lined with myoepithelial cells but their many layers of plump cancer cells had vanished; moreover, the acini no longer contained secretion, detectable amounts of alkaline phosphatase, or carbohydrate.

Estradiol, Progesterone, and Gonadotrophin

Small amounts of an estrogen together with pituitary mammogenic peptide hormones are requisite for the development of prepubertal mammary glands to adult status. The breast remains infantile in the absence of either class of hormones.

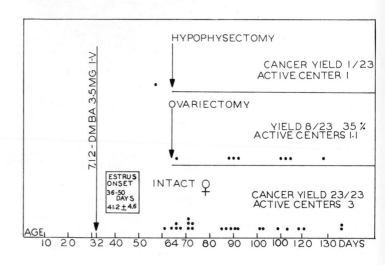

Fig. 7.2. The relative effectiveness of hypophysectomy and ovariectomy in extinction of mammary cancer. At age 32 days, just before the onset of estrus, 7,12-DMBA, 36 mg/kg, was injected intravenously in S-D female rats. At age 64 days, 2 groups of 23 rats were subjected to hypox or ovariex; a group of 23 rats was maintained as intact controls. Autopsy was performed at age 136 days. The day of detection of mammary cancer, subsequently confirmed at autopsy, is indicated by •.

The function of estradiol is to initiate mitosis and promote growth to a mature status; estradiol is not required for carcinogenesis in mature mammary tubules. With regard to hormone-responsive mammary cancer, small amounts of estrogen are permissive for its existence and growth, whereas large amounts destroy the tumors. Progestational steroids accelerate the growth of cancer of the breast. Cantarow, Stasney, and Paschkis 1948 produced mammary cancer by incorporating AAF (0.03%) in the ration of female rats of the Sherman and Wistar strains. Groups of these animals at risk were injected with progesterone thrice weekly. The incidence of mammary cancer was 30% of uninjected controls and 85% of progesterone-treated rats.

The development of mammary cancer following a single feeding of a carcinogen was correlated with the morphology and the specific activity of alkaline phosphatase of the mammary glands of control and hormone-injected rats (Huggins, Moon, and Morii 1962). A solitary dose of 7,12-DMBA (20 mg) was fed to S-D female rats, age 50 days. Always a group of carcinogen-treated rats was kept as controls; all other sets received daily

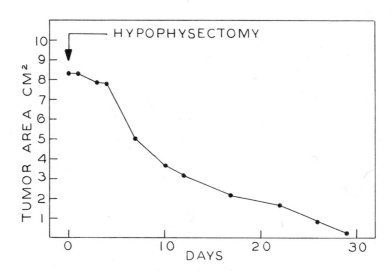

Fig. 7.3. Decrease in surface area of a mammary cancer following hypox.

injections of hormones for only 30 days, from day 15 to day 45; some members of each group were subjected to biopsy of inguinal mammary glands at intervals for histologic and biochemical study. The animals were examined for tumors daily; mammary carcinomas found at autopsy are designated active centers. The experiment was terminated on day 180.

In control animals given a single feeding of 7,12-DMBA but untreated otherwise, the incidence of mammary cancer (table 7.1) was 48 of 48 rats.

1. Estradiol. The appearance of mammary cancer was delayed (table 7.1) in 7,12-DMBA-fed rats injected with estradiol, 20 μg daily, and there were few active centers, but mammary cancer was found in every animal. Estradiol induced considerable growth of lactational type in the mammary glands resulting in a twofold increase of alkaline phosphatase.

2. Progesterone. The daily injection of 4 mg of progesterone resulted in acceleration of the growth of carcinogen-induced mammary cancer; tumors appeared early (table 7.1) and the incidence of mammary cancer was 100%; there were many active centers. The growth of mammary cancer induced by big doses of progesterone mimicked the tumor-accelerating action of pregnancy (table 7.1). Progesterone causes epithelial proliferation of gestational type (p. 109) without lactation. There was a threefold rise of alkaline phosphatase in the mammary glands.

3. Estradiol with progesterone. The daily injection of estradiol, 20 μg, with progesterone, 4 mg, resulted in a pronounced

Table 7.1   Influence of Pregnancy, Ovarian Hormones, and Gonadotrophin on Incidence of Mammary Cancer in Rats Fed 7,12-DMBA

Endocrine status	Number of rats	Rats with cancer		Time of detection of mammary cancer (days)	
		Number	Percent	Range	Mean
Intact controls	48	48	100	27– 72	41 ± 8
Pregnancy	34	34	100	23– 36	30 ± 3
Progesterone, 4 mg*	48	48	100	24– 49	33 ± 5
Estradiol-17β, 20 μg*	31	31	100	60–111	81 ± 14
Progesterone, 4 mg*, plus estradiol-17β, 20 μg*	100	48	48	62–182	124 ± 31
Gonadotrophin, 1 unit*	20	14	70	32–175	90 ± 44

NOTE: All rats were given a single feeding of 20 mg of 7,12-DMBA at age 50 days. One group was bred at age 65 days.
*Groups receiving hormones were injected daily between age 65–95 days; the daily dose of hormones is given. Means with standard deviation ± are given.

decrease in the incidence of mammary cancer; mammary cancer failed to develop in 52% of the rats within 6 months after the carcinogenic dose of 7,12-DMBA, whereas all of their control companions uninjected with hormones had succumbed from massive involvement with mammary cancer.

The combined administration of estradiol and progesterone induced extremely hyperplastic mammary glands of gestational type with a fourfold increase of alkaline phosphatase. The epithelial proliferation was simply an exaggeration of the hyperplasia induced by progesterone alone. Secretion in the acini was minimal. The vaginal cytology was metestrus in type.

It is remarkable that mammary cancer was destroyed by hormones that simultaneously caused exuberant growth of the normal mammary glands of the host.

4. Equine gonadotrophin. One unit (Cartland and Nelson 1937, 1938) was injected daily for 30 days in 20 rats that had received a solitary feeding of 7,12-DMBA at 50 days. Mammary cancer was found in only 14 animals (70%) on day 180 and the appearance of the tumors was retarded (table 7.1).

The big doses of gonadotrophin caused great enlargement of the ovaries, which were cystic. The vaginal cytology was characterized by florid estrus. The mammary glands were hyperplastic and orange in color with epithelial proliferation consisting of solid and luminated tubules. Milk was present in the mammary glands but only in trace amounts. There was a significant reduction in the number of ràts that developed mammary cancer following heavy stimulation of ovarian function with gonadotrophin.

Polyestradiol Phosphate

Fernö et al. 1958 synthesized a series of polymers of phosphoric acid esters of polyphenols and related compounds including estradiol. Polyestradiol phosphate (PEP) is a water-soluble long-lasting estrogen suitable for intravenous injection. (Warning: Pharmaceutical preparations of PEP containing niacinamide administered to humans by intravenous injection may cause a vasomotor reaction.) PEP is stored in the reticuloendothelial cells of liver to form an endocrine depot from which hormones are released slowly but continuously. PEP has enormous unrealized therapeutic potential in the prevention and extinction of mammary cancer.

The early endocrine effects of a big dose of PEP depend on the absence or presence of follicles in the ovary (ovulation) and are manifest in the vaginal cytology. Two types of response to PEP occur:

1. Among rats with no ovarian follicles, that is, prepubertal females and ovariex rats, the response to PEP is uniphasic (fig. 7.4): cornified cells and keratin fibers appear in the vaginal epithelium in $\sim$ 48 hr and persist without interruption for many months.

2. Among rats possessing follicles in the ovary, that is, immature females injected with gonadotrophin for 3 days before PEP and mature females with regular estrus cycles, the response to PEP is triphasic (fig. 7.4): in phase 1, estrus is 1–3 days in duration; in phase 2, metestrus lasts 8–12 days; and in phase 3, uninterrupted estrus persists many months.

During metestrus (phase 2) large corpora lutea are present in the ovary and the mammary glands have exuberant gestational proliferation.

Synthesis of the luteinizing hormone (LH) in the pituitary is normally induced by estrogen. The powerful estrogen, polyestradiol phosphate, causes a surge of synthesis of LH in the anterior lobe of the hypophysis and this peptide hormone in turn produces large corpora lutea in functioning ovarian follicles. The newly formed corpora lutea synthesize progestational steroids, which block estrus, produce metestrus, and cause great mammary hyperplasia. LH maintains the corpora lutea until they undergo attrition, but it cannot produce new ones in the

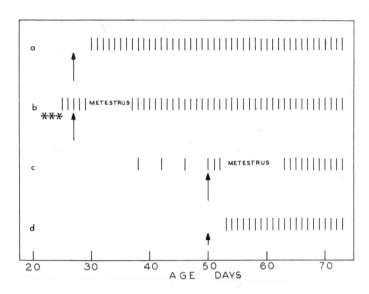

Fig. 7.4. Estrus and metestrus in vaginal smears of rats injected with polyestradiol phosphate (PEP), 50 mg/kg. The response to PEP is uniphasic in females without follicles in the ovary: *a*, infant, age 26 days; *d*, ovariex. The response to PEP is triphasic in ovulating rats: *b*, infant injected with gonadotrophin prior to PEP; *c*, normal adult. ↓, Polyestradiol phosphate injection; *, gonadotrophin injection; |, estrus.

absence of ovarian follicles. After the crop of corpora lutea induced by LH has disappeared, estrus recommences and lactation becomes copious.

Twenty-four S-D rats were subjected to hysterectomy at age 36 days; the ovaries were not disturbed. Regular estrus cycles appeared at age 41–44 days. At age 56 days (day 0) a single feeding of 20 mg of 7,12-DMBA was given by gastric intubation. On day 27 mammary cancer was recognized by palpation in one rat. On day 28, 12 rats received an intravenous injection of 5 mg of PEP (25 mg/kg), whereas 12 control rats were injected with saline. Metestrus was first observed 3 days after the injection of PEP in rats; metestrus lasted for 10.7 ± 2.4 days, and it was followed by estrus, which was present for 4 months thereafter. The experiment terminated on day 124. The incidence of mammary cancer was 12 out of 12 control rats and 0 out of 12 PEP-injected rats.

Proposition 6: Extinction of Mammary Cancer with Estrogen

A single intravenous injection of 5 mg of polyestradiol phosphate is highly effective in destroying mammary cancers induced by carcinogenic hydrocarbons in female rat.

Six female rats of S-D strain were given a single feeding of 20 mg of 7,12-DMBA at age 50 days; the day of feeding the carcinogen is denoted day 0. Mammary carcinoma was observed in every rat in 28–50 days; the mean tumor induction time was 39.3 ± 8 days. Hysterectomy was performed under ether anesthesia; the ovaries were not disturbed.

On day 67, maps of the distribution of the tumors (fig. 7.5) were constructed and it was found that the 6 rats had a total of 22 mammary cancers. On day 67, 5 mg of PEP was injected intravenously. Regression (fig. 7.5) occurred in 4 animals. Necropsy was performed on day 104 with the following findings: 2 rats had a combined total of 3 mammary cancers; 4 rats were cancer-free.

Anti-Estrogens in the Treatment of Mammary Cancer

DeSombre and Arbogast 1974 evaluated an anti-estrogen, C1628 (p. xv) for its ability to effect regression of 7,12-DMBA-induced mammary cancers in S-D rats. In adult females with regular estrus cycles, C1628 (fig. 3.2) abolished the cycles and produced diestrus in the vaginal smear. When the first mammary cancer in an animal had grown to a measurement of 2 cm in any dimension, C1628 was injected subcutaneously 6 times each week until the end of the experiment; the daily dose of C1628 was 1 mg/kg body weight. There resulted a decrease in

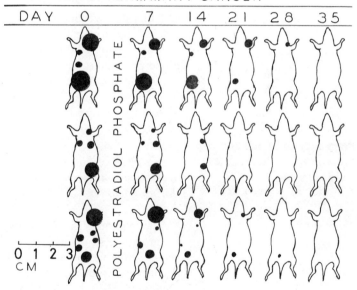

Fig. 7.5. Extinction of mammary cancer in 3 rats; each animal received a single intravenous injection of polyestradiol phosphate, 5 mg.

size of the majority of the tumors and about 25% of the mammary cancers disappeared. The regression of mammary cancers in rats treated with C1628 was often dramatic insofar as large tumors underwent a precipitous decline in size immediately after initiation of the treatment. The effect of C1628 was beneficial but ovariex was more effective in the treatment of mammary cancer than the anti-estrogen was.

In large doses Tamoxifen (p. xvi) is weakly estrogenic; in small quantities it is an anti-estrogen. In the clinical investigation of Ward 1973, Tamoxifen (fig. 3.2) was given by mouth to women with advanced metastatic or recurrent cancer of the breast. A definite response was defined as a reduction in tumor dimensions to half or smaller size persisting for at least 3 months. Responses of this sort were observed in 14 of 35 patients receiving Tamoxifen, 20 mg daily. Lack of toxicity is highly advantageous in anti-cancer drugs in clinical use; undesirable side effects were absent or trivial in the women treated with Tamoxifen.

In the experiments of Fiebig and Schmähl 1978, mammary cancers were induced by intravenous injections of either N-nitrosomethylurea (Gullino, Pettigrew, and Grantham 1975) or 7,12-DMBA. When mammary cancers had developed in the animal, the rat was treated with ovariectomy and Tamoxifen, singly or in combination. Ovariectomy was significantly more effective than Tamoxifen in causing a regression of the cancers. When treatment with Tamoxifen was stopped, the total tumor size of rats receiving this anti-estrogenic compound increased. One of the principal purposes of the experiment was to ascertain if a combined therapy was more effective than ovariectomy alone; the results were negative. The combination of Tamoxifen plus ovariectomy reduced significantly the beneficial result of ovariectomy alone. The adverse effect of Tamoxifen is due to its weakly estrogenic effect.

Pregnancy and Lactation

Proposition 7: Pregnancy and Lactation

The growth of hormone-responsive mammary cancers is accelerated in pregnancy and retarded after parturition and during lactation.

The mammary glands during pregnancy undergo vast changes in growth and function consisting of hyperplasias of two sorts: in the first phase there is gestational proliferation that is exclusively a nonsecretory growth effect preparatory to the secretion of milk; the second phase occurring late in pregnancy is lactational proliferation. Each hyperplasia has a characteristic but opposite effect on hormone-responsive mammary cancer. Gestational proliferation stimulates growth of cancer of the breast, whereas lactational hyperplasia causes regression of experimental mammary cancer.

During gestation mammary glands become greatly enlarged, firm, orange in color: there is a pronounced growth of small mammary tubules devoid of lumina. In the rat gestational proliferation reaches its height on day 15 of pregnancy; thereafter lactational changes occur.

In lactational hyperplasia the mammary acini become greatly enlarged and turgid with milky secretion. In the rat large milk pools are visible through the skin in the gross. Lactational proliferation develops when virgin female rats are injected with large quantities of estradiol-17β (20–100 μg daily).

Bielschowsky 1947 induced mammary cancer in the albino rat by feeding AAF for many months and observed that reproduction had a biphasic effect on the growth of the neoplasms. The growth of mammary cancer was accelerated during pregnancy, whereas its growth was arrested during lactation; in many instances mammary cancer vanishes after parturition.

Dao and Sunderland 1959 found that pregnant rats treated with carcinogenic doses of hydrocarbons were refractory to the induction of cancer of the breast. However, the growth of mammary cancer, which had been elicited before the animal became pregnant, was accelerated during pregnancy. Daily doses of 3-MC (10 mg) were fed to rats for 20 days and the animals were mated 4 days after the termination of carcinogen feeding. Pregnancy increased the development of mammary cancer; the time of appearance of the tumors was accelerated and the number of active centers increased significantly. The tumors rapidly decreased in size following delivery of the babies. Dao and Sunderland 1959 stated that they had not found a single instance in which a tumor failed to regress after parturition.

Huggins, Moon, and Morii 1962 fed a single dose of 7,12-DMBA (20 mg) to S-D rats, age 50 days, and the animals were bred at age 65–70 days. The development of mammary cancer (table 7.1) was accelerated in comparison with that in nonpregnant sisters.

Hypothalamus and Prolactin

The mammalian hypothalamus exerts an inhibitory influence on the synthesis and release of prolactin by the pituitary (Meites 1972a, b); hypothalamic extracts from many species depress the secretion of prolactin by the pituitary and disruption of the pituitary stalk connecting hypothalamus and pituitary results in enhanced release of prolactin.

The release of the prolactin-inhibiting factor (PIF) by the hypothalamus is influenced to a considerable extent by the administration of catecholamines (Meites 1972*a*); an increase in biogenic amines increases release of PIF, reduces prolactin levels, and inhibits the growth of mammary cancer in rat.

Hypothalamic Lesions. Clemens, Welsch, and Meites 1968, by means of stereotaxis, placed lesions in rat's hypothalamus before the induction of mammary cancers with 7,12-DMBA; it was found that the formation and growth of cancers of the breast were retarded by the operation. Welsch 1972 produced lesions in the hypothalamus after inducing mammary cancers with 7,12-DMBA; there resulted an increase of prolactin and accelerated growth of the mammary cancers. It is noteworthy that ovariectomy in the rats with hypothalamic lesions resulted in regression of the mammary cancers, whose growth until that time, had been flourishing.

Sinha, Cooper, and Dao 1973 confirmed the observation that hypothalamic lesions promoted the growth of carcinogen-induced mammary cancer in the rat with an associated increase ($\sim$ fourfold) of plasma prolactin. It was highly significant in these experiments that ovariectomy resulted in rapid and profound regression of mammary cancer despite continuing high levels of prolactin. It would appear that the stimulatory effect of prolactin is related to ovarian function, presumably to an increased activity of corpora lutea, hence in the synthesis of progesterone.

Drugs. When reserpine, a drug that increases the secretion of prolactin, is administered, the development of mammary cancer is accelerated. When drugs such as L-dopa or ergot derivatives, which cause a decrease of prolactin secretion, are administered, the incidence and growth of spontaneous or carcinogen-induced mammary cancer is reduced greatly.

The alkaloid reserpine is a powerful tranquilizer and sedative, which possesses two additional pharmacologic activities: it suppresses ovarian cycles and provokes lactation. Lacassagne and Duplan 1959 found that long-term feeding of reserpine resulted in the accelerated development of spontaneous mammary cancer in mice of the C3H strain; the ovaries of the mice were big and contained large corpora lutea.

Quadri, Kledzik, and Meites 1973 injected rats bearing 7,12-DMBA-induced mammary adenocarcinoma with L-dihydroxyphenylalanine (L-dopa) for 4 weeks; growth of the cancers was retarded and some of the tumors vanished.

In the experiments of Nagasawa and Meites 1970 mammary cancers were induced in S-D rats by a single intravenous injection of 5 mg of 7,12-DMBA. After the tumors reached ~ 1 cm in diameter, the rats were injected for 15 days with ergocornine or for 25 days with iproniazid or dopamine. Ergocornine and iproniazid completely suppressed mammary tumor growth and prevented development of new tumors, whereas in the control and dopamine-treated rats growth of the tumors was considerable and many new tumors appeared. Ergocornine is believed to inhibit mammary cancer by decreasing the secretion of pituitary prolactin.

Prolactin Receptors

Kelly et al. 1974 studied the specific binding of [^{125}I] prolactin in 7,12-DMBA-induced mammary cancer in the rat; the growth rate of the tumors was correlated significantly with the extent of prolactin-binding in the neoplasms. Costlow and McGuire 1977 demonstrated by autoradiography the location of prolactin receptors in 7,12-DMBA-induced mammary cancer; it was found that specific prolactin-binding is confined to the epithelial cells of the neoplasm.

Costlow, Buschow, and McGuire 1976 assayed 7,12-DMBA-induced mammary cancer for prolactin receptors following ovariectomy or hypophysectomy. Actively growing tumors showed a wide range in the binding of prolactin; ovariectomy caused a slight decrease ($\sim 30\%$) in binding regardless of whether the cancers regressed or continued to grow. Hypophysectomy resulted in a prompt decrease ($\sim 90\%$) in prolactin-binding in liver but only a slight lowering in the mammary cancers from the same rat. It would appear that endocrine regulation of prolactin-binding in normal liver is distinctly different from that in neoplastic mammary tissue.

A significant number of human breast cancers respond to endocrine ablations such as ovariectomy, adrenalectomy, and hypophysectomy, and therefore these cancers are considered to be hormone-dependent. The correlation of the remission of breast cancer following endocrine ablation with tumor estrogen-receptor content permits an accurate prognostication for many patients on such therapy so that it is presumed that estrogen is involved in growth regulation of these cancers. However, there are suggestions that prolactin and other peptide hormones may be important in breast cancer. Most of the mammary cancers induced by 7,12-DMBA in the rat regress following treatment with ergot drugs that inhibit prolactin release.

DeSombre et al. 1976 measured the concentrations of estradiol receptors and prolactin receptors in 24 experimental mammary cancers. All of the tumors contained specific estradiol receptors and all but 3 of the tumors contained prolactin receptors; the values for each receptor ranged from very low to relatively high concentrations. All of the tumors with high levels of both estradiol and prolactin receptors regressed following ovariectomy.

8

Induction and Extinction of Leukemia in Rat

In which novel methods are provided for the rapid induction of leukemia in high yields in rat; it is the leukemia machine. During the investigation it was found out that a proportion of the hydrocarbon-induced leukemias could be extinguished by endocrine methods, which included either hypophysectomy or the administration of glucocorticoids. Many of the leukemias that were caused to regress by endocrine interventions did not recur during the life of the animal; the animal was cured of leukemia.

There are many carcinogenic polycyclic aromatic hydrocarbons and aromatic amines that differ widely in chemical structure. Remarkably, with the exception of the azo dyes that evoke liver tumors, all of the carcinogenic compounds elicit an identical pattern of neoplasms. Injected locally, the carcinogens produce fibrosarcoma; when the carcinogens are administered systemically, by mouth or by vein, the most common forms of cancer to arise are leukemia and mammary carcinoma.

Induction of Leukemia

Experiments were carried out on heterozygous rats of two strains with distinctive coat color—albino (S-D) and pigmented (L-E). The two most potent carcinogenic hydrocarbons, 7,12-DMBA and 7,8,12-TMBA, were administered individually in big doses —one rat, one compound. These hydrocarbons are equally carcinogenic but differ considerably in toxicity; in rat 7,8,12-TMBA is much less toxic than 7,12-DMBA is.

It will be recalled that rats of S-D strain are enormously susceptible to the production of mammary cancer by a single dose of 7,12-DMBA or 7,8,12-TMBA, whereas L-E rats are resistant under the stated conditions.

Multiple doses of carcinogenic hydrocarbons are necessary for the induction of leukemia in high yields (> 50% of the animals at risk) in rodents. In L-E rats a single intravenous injection of 7,8,12-TMBA elicited leukemia in 4.3% of the animals and a set of 4 doses of 7,8,12-TMBA evoked leukemia in 82% of the rats (p. 118).

Rats of S-D strain are especially vulnerable to the toxic effects of multiple doses of powerful carcinogens, whereas L-E rats are highly resistant under the stated conditions. S-D rats have a propensity to develop aplastic anemia and a devastating pneumonitis when repeated doses of 7,12-DMBA or 7,8,12-TMBA are given; neither disease is a serious problem in L-E rats under laboratory conditions. The rapid production of leukemia in the highest yields is made possible because of the exceptional tolerance of L-E rats to a series of big doses of 7,8,12-TMBA.

Toxicity of 7,12-DMBA and 7,8,12-TMBA for Rat. The amount of hydrocarbon that killed half of a group (LD_{50}) of rats within 21 days after a single dose was calculated by the probit method of Gaddum (Burn, Finney, and Goodwin 1950). Young rats are more tolerant of 7,12-DMBA than older rats are, and 7,8,12-TMBA is less toxic for rats than 7,12-DMBA is.

1. Single intravenous injection: For L-E rats the LD_{50} for 7,12-DMBA at age 25 days is 73 mg/kg and at age 50 days it is 44 mg/kg. LD_{50} for a single injection of 7,8,12-TMBA is 104 mg/kg at age 50 days.

2. Single feeding: For L-E rats the LD_{50} for 7,12-DMBA at age 50 days is 400 mg/kg; for S-D rats the LD_{50} at age 50 days is 270 mg/kg.

Leukemia in S-D Rat

In the experiments of Shay et al. 1951, 3-methylcholanthrene (2 mg daily, 6 days each week) was tube-fed for many months to albino rats of the Wistar strain; leukemia developed in 14% of the animals. Hartmann et al. 1959 fed a ration containing 0.02% of 2-acetylaminophenanthrene for 2–4 months to albino rats of the Holtzman strain; leukemia was detected in 48% of the animals.

In the experiments of Prigozhina 1962, 7,12-DMBA (1–2 mg semiweekly) was tube-fed to albino rats of the Wistar strain. The incidence of leukemia was 47% and the induction time 2.5–5.0 months; the leukemia was designated "generalized leukosis—erythroblastosis." The gross anatomical findings were remarkably uniform—a huge pale liver with a significantly enlarged spleen occupied the major portion of the peritoneal cavity, whereas thymus and lymph nodes were not involved. The histologic findings were also uniform—a massive diffuse infiltration of the liver with leukemic cells resulted in a sharp reduction in the amount of hepatic structure. The leukemia was transplantable to allogeneic newborn rats, age less than 2 weeks.

Huggins and Grand 1966 administered a set of 6 intravenous injections of 7,12-DMBA (at biweekly intervals starting at age 28 days) to a series of 95 S-D male rats. Each dose of 7,12-DMBA was 35 mg/kg, or 6 mg, whichever amount was smaller. There were 36 early deaths. In 59 survivors the incidence of neoplasms (table 8.1) was leukemia 73% and mammary cancer 69%. It is noteworthy that the hydrocarbon-induced cancers of the breast did not regress following orchiectomy or hypophysectomy; this finding demonstrated that mammary cancers of male rats are hormone-independent.

Table 8.1

Leukemia and Mammary Cancer Evoked in S-D Rats by 6 Intravenous Injections of 7,12-DMBA

Sex	Number of rats	Mammary cancer detected			Leukemia detected		
		Number of rats	Range (days)	Mean (days)	Number of rats	Range (days)	Mean (days)
M	59	41	54–157	93 ± 21	43	62–164	120 ± 29

NOTE: Male rats of S-D stock were given a series of 6 intravenous injections of 7,12-DMBA at intervals of 14 days, starting at age 28 days; the dosage of 7,12-DMBA was 35 mg/kg or 6 mg, whichever was smaller. Means with standard deviation ± are given.

Leukemia in L-E Rat

Spontaneous leukemia is rare in our colony of L-E rats. Among more than 6000 untreated rats of this strain maintained for breeding purposes for 6–12 months, leukemia was observed in one animal—a pregnant female, had developed lymphocytic leukemia.

Proposition 8: Induction of Leukemia by Feeding Carcinogen

Leukemia is elicited in more than half of a series of Long-Evans rats given a set of 8 feedings of a solution of 7,12-dimethylbenz[a]anthracene in sesame oil at biweekly intervals starting during the age period 4–8 weeks. The first dose of 7,12-DMBA is 200 mg/kg; subsequent feedings consist of 10 mg of 7,12-DMBA in 2 ml of sesame oil. Each feeding is given by gastric instillation to a rat under brief ether anesthesia.

Induction of Leukemia by Feeding 7,12-DMBA. Observed for six months were 19 male L-E rats that survived a single feeding of 7,12-DMBA, 325–400 mg; leukemia did not develop in any of these animals.

In the experiments of Huggins, Yoshida, and Bird 1974, 24 consecutive series of L-E rats were given a set of 8 feedings of

7,12-DMBA; each series comprised 12 rats and animals whose initial body weight was less than 50 gm were excluded from the experiment. The first feeding, 200 mg/kg, was given at age 28 days (day 0). Subsequently 7 additional tube-feedings were given at intervals of 14 days; each of these feedings consisted of 10 mg of 7,12-DMBA dissolved in 2 ml of sesame oil.

Leukemia was observed in 1–4 rats in every series before day 52. The neoplasms (table 8.2) were: leukemia, females 82% and males 70%, and mammary carcinoma, females 66% and males 20%.

Table 8.2   Leukemia and Mammary Cancer Evoked in L-E Rats by 8 Feedings of 7,12-DMBA

Sex	Number of rats	Mammary cancer detected			Leukemia detected		
		Number of rats	Range (days)	Mean (days)	Number of rats	Range (days)	Mean (days)
F	56	37	53–117	86.5 ± 16	46	40–162	92.8 ± 31
M	81	16	57–163	102.6 ± 26	57	36–175	92.4 ± 36

NOTE: Rats of L-E stock were fed a series of 8 feedings of 7,12-DMBA at intervals of 14 days starting at age 28 days. The dosage of 7,12-DMBA was: first feeding, 200 mg/kg; each subsequent feeding, 10 mg. Means with standard deviation ± are given.

The day on which leukemia is observed in half of the animals in a series is designated $Leuk_{50}$. In the juvenile rats, $Leuk_{50}$ was day 96 for females and day 106 for males.

Studied histologically were 56 consecutive leukemias produced by series of feedings to juvenile L-E rats. The leukemias were classified as 55 cases of erythroleukemia and 1 case of myelocytic leukemia.

We studied 32 female L-E rats, which were given 8 feedings of DMBA according to the schedule of Proposition 8; the first feeding of the carcinogen was given when the rats were aged 56 days. There were 8 early deaths leaving 24 effective animals. The neoplasms were leukemia in 22 rats (92%), mammary cancer in 9 rats (38%), and ear duct tumors in 2 rats (8%). Leukemia was observed in 76.5 ± 23 days; mammary cancer was found in 88.7 ± 20 days.

Induction of leukemia in L-E rats by a set of feedings of 7,12-DMBA is a serviceable experimental procedure. Leukemia is elicited regularly in every series and yields are high. There is a considerable incidence of mammary cancer, which is significantly greater in females than in males.

There are several advantages in this procedure: animals and materials are readily available from commercial sources; no great technical expertise is demanded; the survival rate is high; and there is freedom from pulmonary infection. There are also two disadvantages: leukemia emerges rather slowly so that Leuk$_{50}$ is day 80–100 and the amounts and the rate of absorption from the gastrointestinal tract are not known.

Induction of Leukemia by Intravenous Injection of 7,12-DMBA. Huggins and Sugiyama 1966 found that multiple injections of 7,12-DMBA elicited leukemia in high yield in L-E rats. Female rats were given a single pulse-injection of 7,12-DMBA, 40 mg/kg, at age 50 days; the incidence of neoplasms was 6.3% with leukemia and no mammary cancer. Companion rats were given 3 injections of 7,12-DMBA (30–40 mg/kg) at age 50, 60, and 70 days; the incidence of neoplasms was 74% with leukemia and 38% with mammary cancer.

Groups of male and female rats were given 4 intravenous injections of 7,12-DMBA at biweekly intervals beginning at age 27 days. Every rat developed leukemia. The animals were sacrificed in the terminal stage of the disease. Survival of the untreated leukemic rats after the first injection of 7,12-DMBA was for males, 132 ± 59 days, and for females, 112 ± 37 days. Mammary cancer developed in 12.5% of the animals of each sex.

The presence of spleen and thymus is not necessary for the induction of erythroleukemia by 7,12-DMBA; erythroleukemia developed rapidly in rats surgically deprived of spleen and thymus prior to a set of leukemogenic doses of 7,12-DMBA.

Induction of Leukemia by Intravenous Injection of 7,8,12-TMBA. The blood of L-E female rats was examined at daily intervals for 14 days following an intravenous injection of 7,8,12-TMBA, 35 mg/kg, at age 50 days. Heparinized blood (0.2 ml) for hematological studies was obtained by cardiac puncture from rats under light ether anesthesia.

The principal findings (table 8.3) were: *i*, increased hemoglobin concentration (days 1–5), *ii*, leukopenia (days 1–7), and *iii*, thrombocytopenia (days 3–14). The leukocyte count on day 3 was $\sim 50\%$ of the preinjection level on day 0; recovery from leukopenia was complete on day 14.

The first dose of 7,8,12-TMBA did not affect normal body growth of the rats but, after second and subsequent doses,

Table 8.3   Hematology of Female L-E Rats Given a Single
                                       Intravenous Injection of 7,8,12-TMBA

Day	Hematocrit (percent)	Hb (percent)	RBC x 10^{-6}/cu mm	Platelets x 10^{-6}/cu mm	WBC/cu mm
0	37.8	10.8 ± 0.4	5.76 ± 0.1	1.05 ± 0.1	$9,817 \pm 497$
1	39.0	11.8 ± 0.3	6.13 ± 0.16	1.08 ± 0.1	$7,287 \pm 338$
3	36.7	12.1 ± 0.3	5.93 ± 0.1	0.91 ± 0.04	$5,009 \pm 420$
5	35.6	11.4 ± 0.3	5.72 ± 0.13	0.89 ± 0.06	$5,155 \pm 432$
7	34.3	10.4 ± 0.2	5.74 ± 0.06	0.97 ± 0.08	$6,573 \pm 875$
10	38.1	11.9 ± 0.3	5.87 ± 0.15	0.75 ± 0.09	$9,249 \pm 998$
14	38.1	11.5 ± 0.4	6.03 ± 0.14	0.38 ± 0.06	$8,532 \pm 1,188$

NOTE: L-E females were given a single intravenous injection of 7,8,12-TMBA, 35 mg/kg, at age 50 days, Blood was obtained by cardiac puncture. The blood examination was made by N. Ueda. Means with standard deviation $\pm$ are given; $n = 8$.

growth was somewhat retarded. Bird 1972 found that repeated doses of hydrocarbon caused a progressive decline in the level of circulating leukocytes and that the "physiological anemia" normally present in immature rats failed to regress.

The effect of the number of doses of carcinogen on the incidence of leukemia was investigated. Female L-E rats were given one or more intravenous injections of 7,8,12-TMBA, 35 mg/kg. Dose 1 was injected at age 50 days; subsequent injections, if appropriate, were given at biweekly intervals and the animals were observed for 6 months.

The incidence (table 8.4) of leukemia was 4.3% with 1 injection, 8.3% with 2 injections, 50% with 3 injections, 82% with 4 injections, and 93% with 5 injections.

Table 8.4   Number of Intravenous Injections of 7,8,12-TMBA
                                       Related to the Incidence of Leukemia

Number of intravenous injections	Number of rats at risk	Incidence of leukemia Number of rats	Percent
1	23	1	4.3
2	12	1	8.3
3	12	6	50
4	11	9	82
5	15	14	93

NOTE: Female rats of L-E strain were given 1–5 intravenous injections of 7,8,12-TMBA 35 mg/kg, at intervals of 14 days beginning at age 50 days.

Proposition 9: Induction
of Leukemia by
Intravenous Carcinogen

Leukemia is elicited rapidly in more than 80% of female rats
of Long-Evans strain given a set of 4 doses of 7,8,12-
trimethylbenz[a]anthracene, 35 mg/kg, by intravenous injection
at biweekly intervals starting at age 50 days.

A series of 4 pulse-injections of 7,8,12-TMBA is highly effective (Huggins, Grand, and Oka 1970) in calling forth leukemia (fig. 8.1) and mammary cancer in female L-E rats. In male rats (table 8.5) leukemia develops preferentially. Leukemia is detected in many animals within 1 month after the first intravenous injection. The predominant leukemia is stem-cell erythroleukemia.

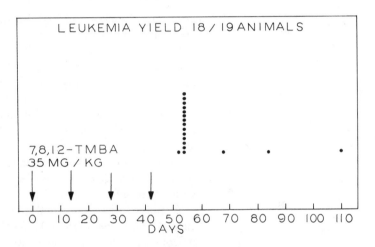

Fig. 8.1. Incidence and day of detection (●) of leukemia in L-E female rats given 4 intravenous injections of TMBA, 35 mg/kg, at biweekly intervals starting at age 50 days.

We studied 10 consecutive series of L-E rats (total 151 animals), which were given a series of 4 intravenous injections of 7,8,12-TMBA, 35 mg/kg, at biweekly intervals starting at age 50 days (day 0). There were 16 deaths (11%) before day 50. Among 135 survivors the incidence of neoplasms (table 8.5) was 88% females and 64% males with leukemia and 16% females and no males with mammary cancer. Leuk$_{50}$ was day 39.

The procedure of Proposition 9 is simple and it is the most efficient method to elicit leukemias with hydrocarbons in any species. There are few early deaths from toxicity. The incidence of leukemia is higher in females than in males. The results have been reproducible through many consecutive series. The regularity and rapidity of induction of leukemia and its extent are awesome. The experimental procedure is useful.

Bird 1972 found that repeated pulse-injections of 7,8,12-TMBA induced severe hypoplasia of bone marrow in L-E rat.

Table 8.5   Leukemia and Mammary Cancer Evoked in L-E Rats
by 4 Intravenous Injections of 7,8,12-TMBA

Sex	Number of rats	Mammary cancer detected			Leukemia detected		
		Number of rats	Range (days)	Mean (days)	Number of rats	Range (days)	Mean (days)
F	69	11	55–100	78.6 ± 16	61	39–134	56.1 ± 21
M	66	0			42	26–101	58.1 ± 12

NOTE: Rats of L-E stock were given 4 intravenous injections of TMBA at intervals of 14 days starting at age 50 days. The dose of 7,8,12-TMBA was 35 mg/kg. Means with standard deviation ± are given.

Leukemia developed in high incidence with invariable involvement of the marrow, whereas the thymus was not implicated.

In the normal adult rat, the bone marrow of the femur is dark red and gelatinous, and it is easily expelled from the marrow cavity. Histologically hematopoietic tissue fills all available marrow spaces in the shaft and epiphyses.

In leukemia, femoral bone marrow is pink or fawn; frequently it is streaked with hemorrhagic areas and is firm; it is less easily expelled from the marrow cavity than normal bone marrow. Leukemic stem cells in bone marrow are identical morphologically with those in the spleen; usually they are admixed with erythroblastic cells.

A characteristic osteopathy develops in rats with leukemia. In the long bones there is thickening of the cortex and marked osseous growth along the endosteal surface of the diaphysis. Many trabeculae of new woven bone form in the bone marrow causing severe narrowing of the marrow cavity (Bird 1972).

Recognition of Leukemia   There are simple but highly effective methods for detecting leukemia in the living rat. They are presented here in the order of utility.

1. Biopsy of liver and spleen is simple and safe. It is of the highest value in diagnosis of leukemias in the rat; in many instances hepatic biopsy is indispensable for recognition of the disease. Because severe thrombocytopenia is frequent in the rats at risk, with consequent danger of fatal hemorrhage during surgical operations, biopsy is not done earlier than 10–12 days after a big dose of carcinogen. In our laboratory hepatic biopsy is performed routinely on day 52–54 after the first dose of carcinogen (day 0) and at biweekly intervals thereafter.

Under ether anesthesia and with asepsis an incision (1 cm) is made in the midline of the upper abdomen. The liver is inspected and the spleen delivered by gentle traction on the greater omentum; cuneiform wedges (50–100 mg) are excised for histological examination; hemostasis is rarely required. The incision is closed in layers with catgut sutures and metallic skin-clips. The procedure takes no more than 1.5–2.0 min.

The signs of leukemia are clear; the liver is big and purple-red; it has a rounded edge and its surface is punctate; the spleen is enlarged, its margins have granular irregularity, and nodules are often present.

Histologic evidence of leukemia in liver (fig. 8.2) and spleen (fig. 8.3) consists of clumps and masses of large, dense baso-philic cells with huge nucleoli. Many mitoses are present.

2. All of our animals are weighed thrice weekly; when the curve of body weight enters a plateau or decreases in animals that have received carcinogen, leukemia is possible. Rats with aplastic anemia lose weight rapidly and the curve of decline is precipitous with a loss of, say, 10–20 g/day. Rats with leukemia lose weight more slowly with a loss of, say, 2–5 g/day. Rats with aplastic anemia have anorexia but with leukemia poly-phagia is commonly present.

3. Physical signs of leukemia in rat include pallor, prominent abdomen, enlarged liver, palpable spleen, superficial lymph nodes which become palpable, dyspnea, and orange-stained fur around urethral meatus.

When leukemic osteopathy (Bird 1972) is present and it is frequent, the rat has a crouched stance with its back arched in a characteristic posture.

4. The microhematocrit is a simple procedure devised for the accurate measurement of the mass of the packed components of the blood; the use of the most slender glass tubing permits quantitative measurement of many components by using the microscope. It is quick and easy routinely to measure the packed mass of thrombocytes, the lymphocytic component, the granu-locytes, and nucleated erythrocytes. The presence of defunct circulating leukocytes is readily observed.

5. Conventional hematologic examination is carried out on blood drawn by cardiac puncture from rodents under brief ether anesthesia.

Method 8.1:
The Microhematocrit

Glass capillary tubing (Cat. No. 46485, Kimble Products, Owens-Illinois, Inc., Toledo, Ohio) has the following

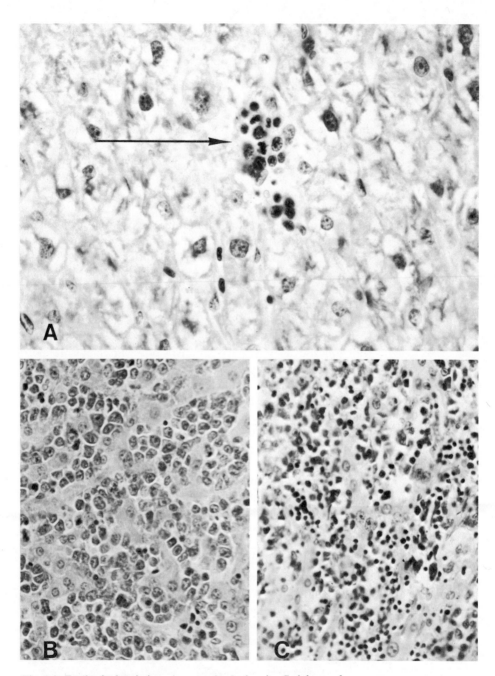

Fig. 8.2. Erythroleukemia in
rat liver: *A*. Arrow points to a
small clump of leukemia cells,
x250. *B*. Advanced stem-cell

erythroleukemia. *C*. Advanced
leukemia with erythroblastic
differentiation. x100.

dimensions: length, 75 mm; external diameter, 0.7–1.0 mm; wall thickness, 0.2 mm; contents $12 \pm 1\mu$l.

Heparinized blood is obtained by cardiac puncture from a rat under light ether anesthesia. The capillary is filled with blood and centrifuged at 12,000 rpm for 5 min; the thickness of the layers of the buffy coat is measured by microscopy (magnification $\times 40$) with an ocular micrometer. The results are expressed in percentage of the length of the capillary (Huggins and Sugiyama 1966; Sugiyama 1973).

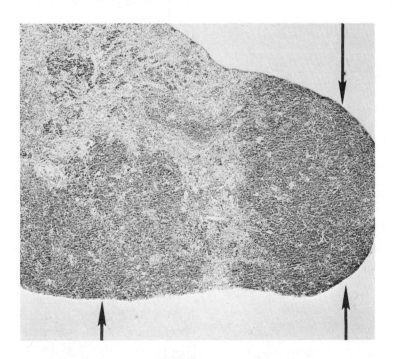

Fig. 8.3. Arrow points to nodules of erythroleukemia in rat spleen. x50.

The Buffy Coat. In the microhematocrit, the buffy coat of rat blood consists of 3 or more distinct layers (Huggins and Sugiyama 1966); the mean thickness of the strata is given in figure 8.4.

Wintrobe 1933 established the use of measurement of the buffy coat as a rough guide to the total leukocyte count. During centrifugation blood cells arrange according to their mass, and the heaviest cells are lowermost (Bessis 1940; Davidson 1960). In rat blood two clearly distinct layers, which we designate B_1 and B_2, are located above the stratum of erythrocytes, R; above these is a pale area, P; occasionally in normal blood a thin layer, U, lies above the P layer at the top of the buffy coat.

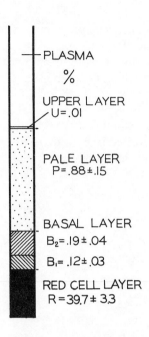

PLASMA

%

UPPER LAYER
U=.01

PALE LAYER
P=.88±.15

BASAL LAYER
B₂=.19±.04

B₁=.12±.03

RED CELL LAYER
R=39.7±3.3

Fig. 8.4. The layers of the buffy coat of blood of normal rats in the microhematocrit; the values are given in percentage.

In the buffy coat the lower basal layer, B_1, consists of granulocytes. The second basal layer, B_2, is composed of mononuclear cells, chiefly lymphocytes. The third layer, P, the thickest stratum of the buffy coat of normal rat, is pale yellow, finely granular, and opaque; it consists of platelets chiefly. The top layer, U, consists of cell "ghosts" and cell fragments but it is not present in every normal blood (Sugiyama 1973).

Important hematologic signs of leukemia are a decrease of the R layer due to anemia, a decrease of the P layer due to thrombocytopenia, and an increase of the U layer associated with increased cell destruction. *In myelogenous leukemia, B_1 layer is increased in thickness; in all other types of leukemia B_2 layer is abnormally thick.*

In aplastic anemia, all of the cell strata in the microhematocrit are decreased in thickness because of pancytopenia.

Transplantation of Blood from Leukemic Donors

Heparinized whole blood, 0.2 ml, obtained by cardiac puncture from a rat with advanced leukemia, was injected into an allogeneic newborn rat, age 24–48 hr; each group consisted of 5–10 rat babes.

1. Intraperitoneal inoculation: Leukemia developed in 85% of the groups and the type of leukemia present in the donor was reproduced in the recipients (Huggins and Sugiyama 1966).

When leukemia was transmitted successfully, the disease was far advanced in 13–38 days.

The liver attained great size in newborn rats inoculated with whole blood from donors with advanced erythroleukemia, sometimes as great as 25% of the weight of the body. The spleen was enlarged in half of the groups, whereas lymph nodes and thymus were never big. Leukemic nodules were found in the omentum in 55% of the groups but peritoneal implants of this sort were not associated with transplantation of blood from leukemias other than erythroleukemia.

Transplantation of whole blood from lymphocytic leukemia of thymic type gave rise to massive involvement of thymus and every lymph node and, to a lesser extent, enlargement of liver and spleen.

Leukemia did not develop in 5 months in newborn rats injected with filtered plasma, 0.2 ml, from leukemic rats.

2. Subcutaneous inoculation: Solid tumors formed at the site of subcutaneous injection of heparinized whole blood, 0.2 ml, from donors with advanced erythroleukemia of rat. These hematosarcomas in the first generation were firm and pale pink in color and they had a characteristic brainlike lobulation (Huggins and Oka 1972). They grew rapidly. On microscopic examination of the hematosarcomas confluent masses of peroxidase-negative leukemic cells were found; mitoses were abundant and normoblasts and erythroblasts were frequent.

3. Reversible conversion of leukemia to hematosarcoma: Simple methods were devised to convert hydrocarbon-induced leukemia cells circulating in the blood of a rat to a solid tumor and *subsequently to return the hematosarcoma to the leukemic form*. The hematosarcomas are advantageous in studying procedures and compounds that cure leukemia since measurement of the size of the tumors is facile. In brief, subcutaneous inoculation of leukemic blood in isogeneic newborn rats gave rise to hematosarcoma; intraperitoneal inoculation of minced hematosarcoma caused leukemia (Huggins and Kuwahara 1967).

Whole blood from a leukemic donor was inoculated in members of a litter of rats, age 0.25–2.0 days; 5 of the recipients were injected subcutaneously and 4 animals were inoculated intraperitoneally. To convert hematosarcoma to leukemia the tumor was excised and minced very fine; it was then diluted with saline so that 0.2 ml contained about 1.5 mg of the mince. Leukemia developed when the suspension (0.2 ml) was injected intraperitoneally; hematosarcoma was propagated by injection subcutaneously.

Types of Hydrocarbon-Induced Leukemia

Huggins and Sugiyama 1966 classified leukemias of the rat according to anatomical characteristics.

1. Erythroleukemia: It is now established that the common hematopoietic target cell for hydrocarbons in rats is a committed erythroid stem cell. For the most part the leukemic cells are arrested at the proerythroblast stage but some of the leukemia cells contain hemoglobin. In the microhematocrit the layer of erythroleukemia cells is pink in color.

Most of the leukemias induced in rats by hydrocarbons are in this category whose outstanding characteristic is the granular and fragile liver which attains huge size—often more than 10% of the body weight. The spleen is big ($>$ 1 gm) in about half of the cases but thymus and lymph nodes are not enlarged.

The hemogram is in the range of that of normal rats until a late stage and then leukocytosis is slight or moderate, usually not exceeding 55,000/mm^3. In the blood very large atypical mononuclear cells (diameter 12–20 μm) are found; mitosis in the circulating leukemia cells is not uncommon.

On histologic examination, large immature tumor cells are found (fig. 8.2) increasingly to invade hepatic sinusoids until the sinusoidal endothelium is completely replaced by them. The large oval nuclei of tumor cells are strongly basophilic. In some cases there is erythroblastic differentiation in the liver. In spleen (fig. 8.3) there is leukemic invasion of the red pulp with lymph follicles preserved until late in the disease. Leukemic infiltration is found constantly in the lymph nodes, the bone marrow, and the middle layer of the adrenal.

2. Myelocytic leukemia: Outstanding characteristics are the high leukocyte count and the typical hemogram of malignant myeloid cells containing granules that are positive for peroxidase and alkaline phosphatase. The liver is normal in size or slightly enlarged. Some of the animals have chloroleukemia, characterized by the green color of thymus, bone marrow, lymph nodes, kidney, and other organs as well as associated mammary carcinoma. On histologic examination, chloroleukemic cells are found in huge clumps in the periportal spaces.

We have encountered three cases of myelocytic leukemia with eosinophilic differentiation. It is of interest that the involvement of the liver is sinusoidal rather than periportal in these cases.

3. Lymphocytic leukemia: A characteristic case had a high leukocyte count with many cells of the lymphocyte series in the hemogram. The spleen was big but often the liver was not enlarged. On histologic examination lymphocytic leukemia in liver was predominantly localized in periportal spaces.

4. Lymphocytic leukemia of the thymic type: The lymphocytic leukemia of T-cells is characterized by a huge thymus, large fused lymph nodes, and a big spleen. This type of lymphocytic leukemia becomes evident because of palpable lymph nodes in the cervical, axillary, and inguinal regions. Dyspnea is present in the terminal stages. Large mononuclear cells, diameter 11 ± 2.8 μm, are prominent in the hemogram.

On histologic examination of the liver, infiltration of lymphoblasts can be seen in the periportal spaces.

In a cumulative series of 134 consecutive cases of leukemia elicited by a series of pulse-injections of 7,8,12-TMBA in rat, Huggins and Oka 1972 classified the types: erythroleukemia 130, myelocytic leukemia 2, and lymphocytic leukemia of the thymic type 2.

Extinction of Leukemia by Endocrine Methods

The regression of leukemia in hormone-responsive cases is dramatic both in the extent and speed of remission. Some lymphocytic leukemias are eliminated by hormone excess following a single massive dose of glucocorticoids. Erythroleukemia is extinguished by hormone-deprival achieved by hypophysectomy.

Glucocorticoid-Induced Regression of Lymphosarcoma. Heilman and Kendall 1944 discovered that cortisone administered to mice bearing a highly malignant transplanted lymphosarcoma brought on a rapid regression of the neoplasm. Dunning 1960 substantiated the beneficial effect of glucocorticoids on transplanted lymphosarcoma of rat.

Huggins and Kuwahara 1967 determined the toxicity of a single dose of a suspension of dexamethasone injected intraperitoneally in L-E rats; LD_{50} was 32.5 mg/kg.

Huggins and Kuwahara 1967 transplanted lymphosarcomas of T-cells subcutaneously in isogeneic L-E rats, age 14 days; the transplants grew rapidly. At age 26 days (day 0) a suspension of dexamethasone, 20 mg/kg, was injected intraperitoneally in half the rats; controls received saline. The experiment was terminated on day 60. The survivors were 2.5% of the controls and 27.5% of the dexamethasone-treated rats.

Regression of Erythroleukemia after Hypophysectomy. The following considerations led us to investigate the effect of hypophysectomy on leukemia: *i*, Van Dyke et al. 1954 observed that the red cell mass decreased to half its original volume after removal of the pituitary; *ii*, Dougherty 1952 observed a diminution in the size of thymus and spleen of rat following hypophysectomy; *iii*, bovine growth hormone increased the size of the atrophic thymus and spleen of hypox rat (Moon et al. 1951); *iv*, there is general hypoplasia of bone marrow (Crafts and Meineke 1959; Gordon 1954; Piliero 1959) accompanied by anemia in the hypox rat; *v*, Moon et al. 1951 noted the absence of spontaneous cancer in hypox rats maintained more than 1 year, whereas lymphosarcoma developed in many rats injected for many months with BGH (Moon et al. 1950); *vi*, the neoplastic response of hypox rat to 7,12-DMBA was significantly decreased (Moon, Li, and Simpson 1956), as manifested by delayed appearance of fibrosarcoma at the site of injection of the hydrocarbon; the administration of BGH restored the carcinogenic response; and *vii*, there is a profound decline in hematocrit and hemoglobin content of the blood after hypophysectomy (fig. 8.5).

Proposition 10: Extinction of Leukemia by Removal of Pituitary

In certain cases hypophysectomy destroys erythroleukemia in rat, and thereby cures the animal.

Huggins and Oka 1972 found out that profound regression followed hypophysectomy in 31% of rats with erythroleukemia induced by a set of pulse-injections of a lipid emulsion of 7,8,12-

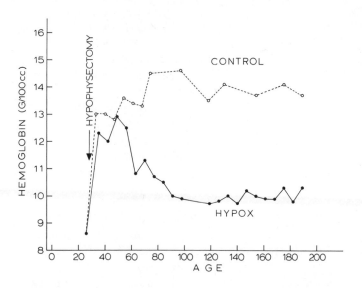

Fig. 8.5. Prolonged decline in hemoglobin content of cardiac blood of rat following hypox.

TMBA in L-E rats. In the favorable cases evidence of improvement following hypophysectomy includes prolongation of life, a decrease of leukemic cells in cardiac blood, diminution or disappearance of histological signs of leukemia in liver and spleen, and complete regression (fig. 8.6) of erythroblastic hematosarcomas in 50% of isogeneic rats that had been inoculated with leukemic blood when they were newborn.

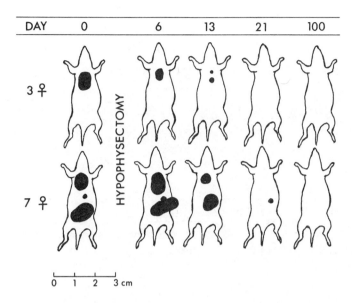

Fig. 8.6. Extinction of hematosarcoma in 2 rats following hypox.

Bentley, Hughes, and Peterson 1974 found that hypophysectomy decreases the susceptibility to leukemia of rats inoculated with the virus of Gross 1961a. Newborn S-D rats were inoculated intraperitoneally with passage A virus and at age 3 weeks half of the animals were subjected to hypophysectomy. The incidence of leukemia 12 weeks after injection of the virus was 37 of 37 unoperated controls and 0 of 11 hypox rats.

Erythroleukemia, Anemia and Erythropoietin

Sugiyama 1971a studied the effect of anemia and plethora on the induction of erythroleukemia by 7,12-DMBA in L-E rats. The incidence of chromosome aberrations in rat bone marrow, examined 6 hr after the administration of 7,12-DMBA, was significantly enhanced by induction of anemia 0–48 hr before the carcinogen treatment and was suppressed by induction of polycythemia. The suppressive influence of polycythemia was reversed by sheep erythropoietin injected shortly before or after the carcinogen injection; this suppressive effect was proportional to the dose of erythropoietin used. These data suggest that erythropoietin is essential to make bone-marrow cells susceptible to chromosome aberrations with 7,12-DMBA. The incidence of carcinogen-induced leukemia was also increased by anemia and suppressed by polycythemia induction.

Selective Cell Destruction in the Adrenal Cortex and Testis Produced by 7,12-DMBA

Members of a class of carcinogens that includes 7,12-DMBA and a few closely related congeners produce distinctive lesions in endocrine glands and hormonal targets of rodents. The effects are big, vivid, and invariable under stated conditions. In rat, lesions include cell destruction in the adrenal glands and testis, but cancer does not arise in these damaged organs nor in the ovary. In mouse, cancer of the ovary is elicited by 7,12-DMBA and 7,8,12-TMBA, whereas adrenal injury is not apparent.

Adrenal Apoplexy

In rat, 7,12-DMBA is a Zauberkugel. A single dose, which need not be hazardous to life, destroys a wide band of the adrenal cortex in the interior of the gland, whereas neighboring cell strata, both superficial and deep, are spared any injury. Massive hemorrhage ensues in the selectively damaged adrenal, whereas bleeding does not occur elsewhere in the rat's body.

This extraordinary destructive effect of 7,12-DMBA is a pharmacologic dissection. It is noteworthy for several reasons: *i*, it is selectively localized; *ii*, it occurs in rat but not in mouse; *iii*, it is dependent on the hormone corticotrophin (ACTH); and *iv*, precise molecular requirements are needed for adrenocorticolysis.

Proposition 11: Production of Adrenal Apoplexy

Female rat of Sprague-Dawley strain, age 50 days, given a single dose of 7,12-dimethylbenz[a]anthracene will develop adrenal apoplexy, which is manifest within 48 hr. The adrenocorticolytic dose is, for intravenous injection, 5 mg (~ 35 mg/kg), and, for intragastric instillation, 30 mg (~ 200 mg/kg). Those females that survive will develop mammary cancer.

The syndrome called adrenal apoplexy, was first described by Waterhouse 1911, as it occurs in the human.

Generally, the disease comes as a flash out of a clear sky. . . . In the classic cases the child wakes up from sleep with a shriek. The temperature rises. . . . The patient now rapidly displays a highly alarming appearance. . . . The body may seem burning hot, while the extremities are icy cold. Simultaneously the blood pressure falls, heart beats and pulse rate become weaker and irregular, respiration shallow and the child passes into a state of shock which leads to death within 4 to 24 hours or 48 hours at the maximum. [Friderichsen 1955]

Hydrocarbon-Induced Adrenal Destruction

Huggins, Grand, and Brillantes 1961 discovered that a single feeding of a massive but generally tolerable quantity of any of a small number of hydrocarbons induced cancer of the breast in every rat under specific conditions; of these compounds 7,12-DMBA was especially effective as a mammary carcinogen (Huggins and Yang 1962). It was soon found out that 7,12-DMBA and its congeners possess unique properties that set them apart from the generality of other powerful hydrocarbons including 3-MC, BP, AAF, and others. Among the distinctive attributes of the 7,12-DMBA group is the capacity to destroy specifically and selectively the middle layer of the adrenal glands of adult rat. The vulnerable layer comprises zona fasciculata and zona reticularis; nonvulnerable regions of the adrenal are zona glomerulosa and the adrenal medulla. The rat with adrenal apoplexy does not appear ill and needs no supportive therapy with corticosteroids or saline drink because the aldosterone-secreting cells of zona glomerulosa are not injured and as a consequence the rat does not develop adrenal insufficiency.

We came upon the adrenocorticolytic property of the 7,12-DMBA group in adult rats in studies on experimental cancer of the breast at the lab bench. At routine examination of rats bearing mammary cancer, which had been elicited by a single feeding of 7,12-DMBA given a few weeks earlier to adult animals, it was observed that most of the adrenals contained palpable masses resembling grains of sand; the adrenal stones had the crystal structure of hydroxypatite. The adrenals of adult rats with mammary cancer, evoked by carcinogens other than members of the 7,12-DMBA group, were not calcified. Retrospective studies were initiated immediately. Soon it was apparent that hemorrhage of gross proportions (fig. 9.1) occurred in all adult rats in the adrenal soon after the animals had been given a large dose of 7,12-DMBA (Huggins and Morii 1961). The destruction was not immediate but occurred 24–33 hrs after admin-

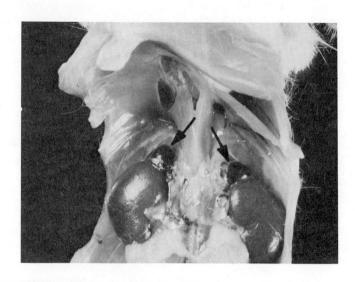

Fig. 9.1. Bilateral adrenal
apoplexy (arrows) in rat, age 53
days, on day 3 following a
single feeding of 30 mg
of DMBA.

istering the carcinogen. The lesion developed soon after mitosis
had taken place in the adrenal. It was remarkable that 7,12-
DMBA did not injure the adrenal glands of juvenile rats or of
mice of any age.

Production and Assay of Adrenal Apoplexy. By definition,
adrenal apoplexy is hemorrhage visible in the gross in the suprarenal glands. In early stages adrenal apoplexy is manifest as one
or several small patches of extravasated blood visible to the
unaided eye on the surface of the gland; these patches coalesce
to form a large, turgid, brilliant red structure reminiscent of a
red light in the dark. Edema is commonly found in the retro-
peritoneal space but periadrenal hemorrhage seldom is observed.

Young adult S-D female rats, age $\sim$ 50 days, were the prototype for our experiments, in which a single dose of 7,12-
DMBA was given. The techniques for the production of adrenal
damage are simple (method 9.1). The corticolytic agent may
be administered by gastric instillation or intravenous injection.

Method 9.1: Production
of Adrenal Apoplexy

The experimental animals were intact female S-D rats, age
47–51 days, weight 146–87 g. The adrenocorticolytic agent
was 7,12-DMBA administered as a single feeding or intravenous
injection (Huggins and Morii 1961). There were 6–8 rats
in each group. The compound was given at 0 hr; adrenals were
harvested at +72 hr.

Intragastric instillation: The rat was anesthetized briefly.

A single dose of 30 mg of 7,12-DMBA (200 mg/kg) dissolved in 2 ml of sesame oil was fed by gastric tube.

Intravenous injection: A single dose of 5 mg of 7,12-DMBA ($\sim$ 35 mg/kg) in 1 ml of a lipid emulsion (Schurr 1969) was injected in a caudal vein.

Just before autopsy the rat was anesthetized with ether and blood was drawn by cardiac puncture for determination of corticosterone levels in the plasma by the fluorometric method of Guillemin et al. 1959. The rat was decapitated; the adrenals were weighed on a torsion balance. The left adrenal was homogenized in ice-cold 0.15M NaCl-3mM NaHCO$_3$ (2 ml) in a Polytron homogenizer for three 10-second bursts at the maximum setting. Homogenates were centrifuged at 12,000 $\times$ g for 15 min at 2°; the supernatant was removed for the assays; blood pigments were estimated by the method of Huggins and Pataki 1965. The right adrenal was prepared for histologic examination or determination of its corticosterone content (Guillemin et al. 1959).

Adult female rats injected with 7,12-DMBA, 18 mg/kg or more, always developed massive adrenal apoplexy (fig. 9.1), but adrenal insufficiency did not ensue. The first abnormalities were detected at 24 hr; the adrenals were brown instead of the customary yellow; the circulation in the sinusoids was similar to that of untreated sisters and the endothelium of the adrenal sinusoids was phagocytic, appearing to be undamaged. Significantly, at 24 hr moderate numbers of shrunken, disrupted, hormone-secretory cells were found despite the apparent integrity of the vascular apparatus. At 30 hr one-third of the adrenals contained large hemorrhages. At 48 hr adrenal apoplexy was full blown; all the adrenals were large, scarlet, and distended with blood.

There were great decreases in levels of corticosterone in adrenal and blood (Huggins, Deuel, and Fukunishi 1963). On histological examination it was found that the entire middle zone had been destroyed (fig. 9.2), but zona glomerulosa and adrenal medulla were usually not injured. In a few adrenals that were tense with hemorrhage the medulla was damaged and small patches of gangrene involved zona glomerulosa; these effects can be attributed to pressure necrosis. At 11 days regeneration of adrenal cortex from zona glomerulsa was well underway and calcification had begun in the necrotic tissue. The adrenal stones remained in both glands for more than 18 months—stigmata of earlier selective destruction.

Corticotrophin-Dependence of Adrenal Apoplexy

The principal steroids in rat adrenal are corticosterone and 11-dehydrocorticosterone (Bush 1953; Morii and Huggins 1962).

The adrenal cortex must be in a susceptible state in order for damage by 7,12-DMBA to be effected. Recent stimulation by considerable amounts of ACTH is necessary for corticolysis to occur; accordingly the effect is hormone-dependent. Spared from injury by 7,12-DMBA are the adrenals of infant rats and those of adults some 3 or more weeks after hypophysectomy.

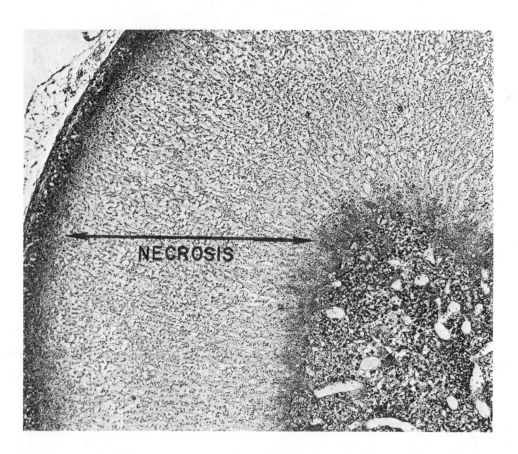

NECROSIS

Fig. 9.2. On day 3, after a single feeding of 30 mg of 7,12-DMBA, complete necrosis of inner zones of adrenal cortex is found. x60.

In S-D rats puberty is an endocrine change that takes place gradually between the ages of 30 and 45 days and remarkable biochemical effects develop in the adrenals during this phase of life. Striking changes are: *i*, a profound decline in the concentration of isocitric dehydrogenase (Huggins and Morii 1961); *ii*, a pronounced rise in the level of corticosterone (Morii and

Huggins 1962); and *iii*, development of vulnerability to 7,12-DMBA.

A single feeding of 30 mg of 7,12-DMBA was provided to members of groups of rats age 25–50 days; the adrenals were harvested at +72 hr. Adrenal necrosis and hemorrhage did not occur in animals age 25–30 days but were found in every rat 50 days old.

ACTH renders the adrenal cortex of infant rats susceptible to destruction by 7,12-DMBA, whereas BGH was ineffective in this regard (table 9.1). Rats were injected with ACTH, 8 I.U. daily, from age 20 to 26 days and then 30 mg of 7,12-DMBA was fed; 72 hr later the adrenals were collected. All the ACTH-treated rats that had been fed 7,12-DMBA developed adrenal apoplexy; none of the adrenals of animals that had received either ACTH or 7,12-DMBA alone was damaged.

Table 9.1　　　　　　ACTH-Induced Vulnerability of Adrenal Cortex of Juvenile Rats to Damage by 7,12-DMBA

Number of rats	ACTH 8 units/day	BGH 0.25 mg/day	Deaths	Rats with adrenal apoplexy
12	No	No	0	0/12
13	No	Yes	1	0/12
15	Yes	No	4	10/11

NOTE: Pituitary peptides (ACTH or BGH) were injected daily from age 20 to 26 days; all rats were fed 30 mg of 7,12-DMBA at age 27 days. The adrenals were harvested at age 30 days.

In the experiments of Morii and Huggins 1962, 5 mg of 7,12-DMBA was injected in a caudal vein of female rats that had been hypophysectomized at age 50 days. Adrenal apoplexy was observed in all of the animals injected with 7,12-DMBA 2 hr to 7 days after hypox and in no animal 14 to 21 days after removal of the pituitary.

The injection of ACTH, 8 units daily for 7 days beginning 21 days after hypophysectomy (day 0), restored the adrenal to the susceptible state wherein 7,12-DMBA induced necrosis and hemorrhage in the glands; 7,12-DMBA was injected on day 7 and autopsy was on day 10. It is noteworthy that adrenal injury was not observed in a comparable group differing only insofar as BGH, 0.25 mg, replaced ACTH (table 9.1).

Adrenal damage is not the result of an interaction between ACTH and 7,12-DMBA. Corticosterone content of the adrenals was measured by a fluorometric technique (Guillemin et al. 1959) and expressed in μg/g; in intact female rats, age 50 days, the corticosterone level was 118 ± 14, whereas in sisters 3 days after hypophysectomy it was 6.6 ± 1. Adrenal apoplexy was induced by 7,12-DMBA in these hypox (3 days) rats despite the low content of adrenal corticosterone. It is inferred (Huggins and Sugiyama 1965) that the preliminary stimulation by ACTH, which is necessary for production of this sort of adrenal apoplexy, is concerned with ACTH-induced maturity of the adrenal's middle layer rather than with corticosterone itself.

Molecular Structure of Corticolytic Hydrocarbons

Solutions of the test compounds were given to female S-D rats, age 50 days, at 0 hr; the adrenals were harvested at $+72$ hr and processed as in method 9.1.

Intragastric Instillation: Whereas a single feeding of 7,12-DMBA (30 mg) by intragastric instillation (Huggins and Morii 1961) induced adrenal apoplexy in 10 of 10 rats, adrenal damage did not occur following a feeding (30 mg) of 1,12-DMBA, 3,9-DMBA, or 6,8-DMBA. A feeding of the transannular peroxide of 7,12-DMBA (50 mg) did not cause injury to the adrenals. A sample of 7,12-dimethylbenz[a]anthracene-16d was tested; our compound had greater than 95% of its hydrogen atoms replaced by deuterium in both ring and side chain sites; the compound (50 mg) produced adrenal apoplexy in 4 of 10 animals. Pathologic changes in the adrenals were not elicited by 7,12-diethylbenz[a]anthracene (100 mg).

Five compounds that have large representation as components in the 7,12-DMBA molecule did not cause pathologic changes in the adrenals. The compounds, inactive in this regard, were 1,4-dimethylphenanthrene, 9,10-dimethylanthracene, benz[a]anthracene, 7-methyl-, and 12-methylbenz[a]anthracene.

Five strongly carcinogenic compounds did not cause adrenal apoplexy. These aromatics were 3-MC, BP, 4-dimethylaminostilbene, 4-nitroquinoline-N-oxide, and AAF. All of these compounds evoke cancer locally when painted on skin or injected in leg muscle in certain species of rodents. All of these hydrocarbons when fed to female rat on a single occasion under stated conditions induce mammary cancer selectively (Huggins 1962).

In rat, a single feeding of a big dose of 7,12-DMBA caused diarrhea, severe leukopenia, and transitory loss of weight. In addition, there was a profound decline (fig. 9.3) in the level of alkaline phosphatase in blood plasma to low levels because of

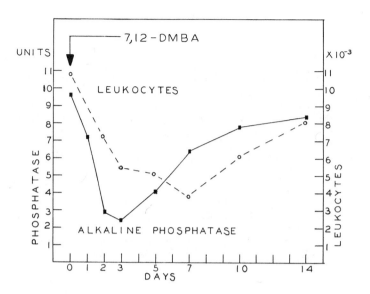

Fig. 9.3. Following a single feeding of 30 mg of 7,12-DMBA at day 0, there was a pronounced decline in plasma alkaline phosphatase and circulating leukocytes (per 1 mm^3). Huggins and Morii 1961.

the failure to absorb unsaturated lipids from the alimentary tract (Huggins and Morii 1961).

Intravenous Injection. Ten compounds are known to cause adrenal apoplexy following intravenous injection (table 9.2). All of the corticolytic hydrocarbons are derivatives of benz[a]anthracene. All possess two side chains at, respectively, C_7 and C_{12}. In every compound the side chain at position 12 is a methyl group; at position 7 several sorts of side chains are permissible for the induction of corticolysis, including alkyl, methoxymethyl, formyl, or hydroxymethyl groups (Huggins, Morii, and Pataki 1969). It is noteworthy that 6,7,12-TMBA and 7,8,12-TMBA are corticolytic, whereas 5,7,12-TMBA and 6,8,12-TMBA are inactive in this regard (Huggins, Grand, and Oka 1970). The most potent corticolytic agent is 7-hydroxymethyl-12-methylbenz[a]anthracene, followed in rank by 7,12-DMBA (Boyland, Sims, and Huggins 1965).

Boyland and Sims 1965 found that the main products of metabolism of 7,12-dimethylbenz[a]anthracene are the isomeric monohydroxymethyl derivatives. It is noteworthy that 7-hydroxymethyl-12-methyl-BA was the most active corticolytic agent in the series, whereas 7-methyl-12-hydroxymethyl-BA did not injure the adrenal cortex.

The entire ring system in 7,12-DMBA and the methyl group at C_{12} provide a nonpolar site for attachment in adrenal tissue by charge transfer or hydrophobic bonding. The hydroxyl group of the C_7 side chain attached to the *meso*-anthracene region of

Table 9.2   Adrenocorticolytic Hydrocarbons

Compound	Melting point	Dose mg	Adrenal hemorrhage
7-Hydroxymethyl-12-MBA	164–166	2	14/14
7,12-DMBA	122–123	4	16/16
7-Formyl-12-MBA	113–114	5	6/8
7-(1-Hydroxyethyl)-12-MBA	124–126	5	6/6
7-(2-Hydroxyethyl)-12-MBA	125–128	5	4/6
7-Methoxymethyl-12-MBA	119–121	5	14/14
7,8,12-TMBA	178.5–179.5	7.5	8/8
6,7,12-TMBA	126–127	7.5	8/8
7-Et-12-MBA	69.5–70.5	15	10/16
7-(1-Hydroxy-*n*-propyl)-12-MBA	69–69.5	15	2/6

NOTE: S-D female rats, age 47–51 days, received a single injection intravenously of a homogenized hydrocarbon and the adrenals were harvested 72 hr. later.

the molecule provides a site for polar hydrophilic attachment presumably by hydrogen bonding.

Prevention of Adrenal Damage by Enzyme Inhibitors

When it was found that 7,12-DMBA produces massive but selective corticolysis (Huggins and Morii 1961) in adult rat, it was postulated that one of the parameters in its pathogenesis was the geometric two-dimensional similarity of the carcinogen to corticosteroids. Compounds that inhibit the introduction of hydroxyl groups into steroids have been found to prevent 7,12-DMBA-induced adrenal destruction.

Currie, Helfenstein, and Young 1962 investigated the effect of 2-methyl-1,2-*bis*-(3-pyridyl)-1-propanone (Metyrapone), a compound that inhibits 11β-steroid hydroxylation and thereby interferes with the synthesis of corticosterone and cortisol; it was found that Metyrapone completely prevented 7,12-DMBA-induced adrenal necrosis. It has been shown that 7-hydroxymethyl-12-MBA is two times more potent than 7,12-DMBA in its adrenocorticolytic action (table 9.2). Wheatley et al. 1966 found that Metyrapone completely protected the adrenal glands against the corticolytic action of 7-hydroxymethyl-12-MBA. Jellinck, Garland, and McRitchie 1968 found that 3-(1,2,3,4-tetrahydro-1-oxo,2-naphthyl)-pyridine (Ciba SU-9055), which is an inhibitor of 17α-steroid hydroxylation, also protects the adrenals against 7,12-DMBA-induced adrenal necrosis in spite of the fact that rat adrenal does not synthesize 17α-hydroxylated corticosteroids.

Spironolactone is a hormonally inactive steroid lactone that inhibits the effect of aldosterone on the renal tubules thus increasing sodium excretion and causing potassium retention. Kovacs and Somogyi 1969 found that spironolactone protects the rat against 7,12-DMBA-induced adrenal necrosis.

Selective Destruction in Testis

Proposition 12: Selective Destructio in Testis

The germinal epithelium of the testis is severely damaged when a male rat, age 25 days, is given a single intravenous injection of 2 mg of 7,12-dimethylbenz[a]anthracene. The primary sites of destruction in the tubules of the testis are exclusively those cells actively synthesizing DNA, whereas nonsynthesizing cells are spared from injury.

Anatomical Effects. In the experiments of Ford and Huggins 1963, 70 male S-D rats, age 25 days and mean weight 65 gm, were given a single intravenous injection of 2 mg of 7,12-DMBA ($\sim$ 30 mg/kg); the day of injection is denoted day 0. The control rats were untreated.

Uninjected control rats had a progressive increment of testis weight (fig. 9.4) between age 25 and 100 days. At age 25 days the seminiferous epithelium consisted of 3 classes of cells: sertoli cells, spermatogonia, and spermatocytes; spermatids and spermatozoa were absent. At age 40 days the first spermatozoa were found.

In the rats injected with 7,12-DMBA at age 25 days, the testis increased in mass (fig. 9.4) for 15 days (age 40 days) when the curve of testis weight entered a plateau lasting for 25 days. Thereafter there ensued a progressive increment of testis weight. The average weights of testis of injected and uninjected rats were similar at about day 75 (age 100 days).

In testis, the primary site of damage is a selective row of germinal epithelial cells near the basement membrane of the tubule; the damaged cells are spermatogonia and resting primary spermatocytes. The selective destruction by 7,12-DMBA of diploid cells in testis during synthesis of DNA is similar to the effect of a heavy dose of radiation on rat testis. In a classic study Regaud and Blanc 1906 found that x-rays destroyed spermatogonia (diploid cells) whereas spermatozoa (haploid cells) were uninjured.

The lesions in testis of rats injected with 7,12-DMBA at age 25 days were apparent on days 1–3 when a decrease in number

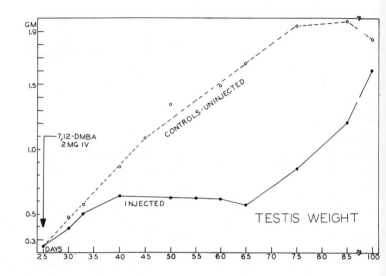

Fig. 9.4. Growth of testis in rats given an intravenous injection of 2 mg of 7,12-DMBA at age 25 days related to that of uninjected controls.

of spermatogonia was observed. On day 6, the number of resting and pachytene spermatocytes was smaller than in the controls. On days 8–11 the "necklace" of densely staining spermatocytes, near the basal cells, disappeared. On day 20 all of the seminiferous tubules were abnormal. There was an increase of spermatogonia but a marked depletion of primary spermatocytes and early spermatids; late-stage spermatids and spermatozoa were present. The greatest atrophy was evident on day 40, but subsequently rather rapid recovery ensued. The testis had returned to an essentially normal state 75 days after a single intravenous injection of 7,12-DMBA.

In rats injected intravenously with a single dose of 2 mg of 7,12-DMBA at age 25 days, the growth of the ventral prostate was similar to that in uninjected brothers; this signified that the interstitial cells of the testis had not been damaged by 7,12-DMBA.

Radioactivity. Incorporation of tritium-labeled thymidine into cellular constituents indicates synthesis of DNA; radioautography is essential for the histochemical localization of this process of DNA replication. In the seminiferous epithelium spermatogonia and resting primary spermatocytes (fig. 9.5) are the only cells that incorporate [³H]TdR (Clermont, Leblond, and Messier 1959; Monesi 1962; Jensen, Ford, and Huggins 1963). These are precisely the cells destroyed by 7,12-DMBA; the subsequent atrophy, and it is of a very high grade, is due to the suppression of these cells, which are the progenitors of the haploid cells, which include spermatids and spermatozoa. The uninjured haploid cells continue their differentiation unchecked so that spermatozoa are formed in profusion despite severe damage by 7,12-DMBA in the prepuberal testis of a rat. For this reason the injured testis of a rat, age 25 days, continues to increase in mass for ~ 2 weeks after an injection of 7,12-DMBA until a plateau of weight is reached.

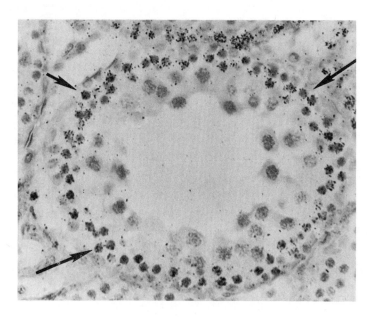

Fig. 9.5. Radioautograph of testis of rat 21 hr after an injection of [³H]TdR. Tritium is present in spermatogonia (arrows) and resting spermatocytes but in no other cell in the testis tubule.

The testis has a high mitotic index characterized by rapid renewal of cells with easily recognizable stages of differentiation (Leblond and Clermont 1952). There is a remarkable synchrony of mitosis (hence of DNA replication) in spermatogonia in individual tubules of testis. In the rat as in the mouse in a cross section of the seminiferous tubules, either all of the cells of the basal layer are labeled or none of this group of cells incorporate tritiated thymidine in that cross section (Edwards and Klein 1961). Spermatogonia that fail to incorporate [³H]-TdR in concert with the generality of their mates are designated asynchronous. Nearly all of the spermatogonia and resting primary spermatocytes are destroyed by a single intravenous injection of 7,12-DMBA (30 mg/kg). Undamaged are asynchronous diploid cells and the haploid cells. In brief, cells that were not incorporating [³H]TdR escaped injury from cell-destructive doses of 7,12-DMBA.

The administration of 7,12-DMBA 4 hr *prior* to the injection of tritium-labeled thymidine considerably depresses the incorporation of tritium into rat testis, intestine, and adrenal (Jensen, Ford, and Huggins 1963). Recovery from the effect of 7,12-DMBA occurs in intestine within 48 hr but in testis and adrenal the inhibitory effect of a single dose of 7,12-DMBA persists for many days. Fractionation of the testis demonstrated that the decrease in tritium content is associated entirely with the washed perchloric acid-insoluble fraction, which is predominantly DNA. The injection of 7,12-DMBA 4 hr *after* [³H]TdR did not depress the incorporation of tritium (DNA-synthesis) in ileum or testis.

From the foregoing experiments it is clear that: *i*, 7,12-DMBA has a striking ability to depress the rapid incorporation of tritiated thymidine into at least 3 tissues, adrenal, intestine, and testis; *ii*, under the conditions of the experiment the depression of synthesis of DNA is massive but not total; *iii*, time *t* is required for 7,12-DMBA to react with cells before its full effect in depressing replication of DNA is realized (the relation is 1 hr $< t <$ 4 hr); and *iv*, 7,12-DMBA causes lesions in cells exclusively during replication of deoxyribonucleic acid.

It would appear that the multiplicity of biological effects of 7,12-DMBA causing cancer and destroying cells are different manifestations of a common effect on nucleic acid formation and integrity.

10

Prevention of Hydrocarbon-Induced Leukemia and Mammary Cancer

Many aromatic hydrocarbons, despite a wide disparity in molecular structure, possess in common the ability to induce protection against the most powerful cancer-producing chemical substances, including 3'Me-DAB, AAF, 7,12-DMBA, 7,8,12-TMBA, and other carcinogens. The protection includes prevention of mammary cancer and leukemia, and preservation of life when rat is given what would otherwise be an overwhelming dose of carcinogen, one that kills the unprotected mates. The experiments on carcinogen protection are simple and quantitative and have sharp and unequivocal end points.

The protector increases hepatic enzymes which inactivate the carcinogen, rendering it innocuous. Because protein synthesis is a prerequisite to protection, it is mandatory that the inducer of protection be given at least 2 hr prior to the challenging carcinogen; otherwise protection does not ensue. Under stated conditions a small dose of the carcinogen induces enzymes that protect against a large amount of itself—the cancer-producing substance is self-protective: 7,12-DMBA prevents damage from 7,12-DMBA (Dao and Tanaka 1963b).

Azo dyes, of which 1-(p-phenylazo-phenylazo)-2-naphthol (Sudan III) is a prototype, are highly effective inducers of protection. Sudan III has special advantages; it protects in minute amounts and is effective when administered via the alimentary tract; it is not toxic; it does not elicit sarcoma when it is injected in leg muscle of rat; it is highly colored so that small amounts in tissues are easily recognized.

Sudan III and related naphthalene dyes have been used for many decades as cosmetics (lipstick) and, it would appear, do not cause cancer in the human. Sudan III can protect against many cancer-producing substances present in our diet and environment.

We have found three simple methods to be especially useful as rapid screening procedures in the identification and evaluation of protectors against carcinogens. These are: *i*, prevention of the massive hemorrhage in the adrenal cortex invariably produced by 7,12-DMBA under stated conditions (p. 130); *ii*, measurement of activity of a soluble enzyme, menadione reductase (EC 1.6.99.2), in the cytosol of liver homogenate; and *iii*, prevention of death in rats given a massive dose of 7,12-DMBA.

Prevention of Azo Dye-Induced Liver Tumors

Richardson and Cunningham 1951 found that trace amounts of the strong carcinogen 3-MC prevented the formation of liver tumors in rat fed a highly potent hepatic carcinogen, 3′-methyl-4-dimethylaminoazobenzene; these workers referred to their important finding as an "accidental" discovery. Two groups of rats, control and experimental, were fed 3′-Me-DAB, incorporated in the basal ration, for many weeks. In the control groups liver tumors developed in 100% of the rats in 15–29 weeks. The experimental group, fed a similar ration containing 3′-Me-DAB, received additionally each week an instillation of 60 μg of 3-MC in the vagina. In the experimental group after 33 weeks of treatment with the two carcinogens, dietary and topical, liver cancer was found in only 17% of the animals.

Subsequently it was observed that the occurrence of liver tumors caused by feeding 3′-Me-DAB was inhibited by several other polycyclic aromatic hydrocarbons incorporated in the ration. The incidence of hepatic neoplasms was lessened significantly when the basal ration containing azo dye was supplemented further with any of the following hydrocarbons: noncarcinogenic BA or carcinogenic BP, DBA, 3-MC (Miller et al. 1952; Richardson et al. 1952).

In extending this work, Miller, MacDonald, and Miller 1954 found that 3-MC strongly inhibited the carcinogenic activity of 2-acetylaminofluorene (AAF) when both carcinogens were added to the basal ration. In rats fed AAF (1.3 mM/kg diet) as the sole additive for 16 weeks, the incidence of tumors was 73% hepatic tumors in males and 73% mammary cancer in females. In rats fed AAF *plus* 3-MC (0.13 mM/kg diet) the incidence of tumors was no hepatic tumors in males and 14% mammary cancer in females.

Conney, Miller, and Miller 1956 found that the activity of rat liver homogenates to demethylate 3-methyl-4-monomethyl-aminoazobenzene (N-demethylase) and to reduce the azo linkage of 4-dimethylaminoazobenzene (reductase) was increased about threefold by 3-MC injected 24 hr prior to assay.

The intraperitoneal injection of 1.86 μM of potent carcinogens BP, DBA, or 3-MC caused a large increase in the synthesis of hepatic demethylase in weanling rats within 24 hr. The increase in enzyme protein was parallel to the ability of the carcinogens to prevent liver tumors in rats when added at low levels to rations containing the strong hepatic carcinogen 3'-Me-DAB.

Conney, Miller, and Miller 1956 studied the effects of amino acid antagonists on induction of hepatic enzymes. Ethionine 0.3 mM (ca. 50 mg) injected into rats 1 hr prior to 3-MC prevented the rise of hepatic N-demethylase but did not modify the activity of the basal levels of preformed enzyme. Methionine did not alter the rate of enzyme induction by 3-MC. The inhibitory effect of ethionine (blocking) on enzyme induction was prevented by concurrent injection of an equimolar amount of methionine (counterblocking); glycine and alanine were ineffective as countermeasures to ethionine inhibition.

Arcos, Conney, and Buu-Hoi 1961 found a relationship between the size of the enzyme inducer and its activity. Polycyclic aromatic hydrocarbons of an optimal molecular size of 85–150 Å² induce the synthesis of hepatic microsome-bound enzymes that demethylate azo dyes and inactivate the muscle relaxant zoxazolamine (2-amino-5-chlorobenzoxazole) by hydroxylation. However, certain compounds whose molecular size fell within this favorable encumbrance area were inactive as enzyme inducers.

Drug-Metabolizing Enzymes

The enzymes that detoxify foreign compounds are of three sorts: *i*, enzymes engaged in biosynthesis or ascorbic acid; *ii*, insoluble enzymes, absent from the cytosol, which are bound to microsomes or the membranes of the smooth endoplasmic reticulum; *iii*, soluble enzymes, including menadione reductase; the three biosynthetic systems rise and fall in unison. Among the most powerful inducers of the drug-metabolizing enzymes are phenobarbital, 3-MC, and azo dyes.

1. Ascorbic Acid Biosynthesis: Longenecker, Fricke, and King 1940 found that the excretion of ascorbic acid by albino rats was augmented greatly by a series of compounds widely used as nerve depressants. The addition of sodium phenobarbital to the ration soon raised the daily excretion of ascorbate from 0.2 to 10 mg daily and individual animals excreted as much as 50–60 mg/day. Conney and Burns 1959 found that 3-MC is a potent stimulator of ascorbate biosynthesis via the glucuronic-gulonic acid pathway. Touster, Hester, and Siler

1960 found that ethionine incorporated in the ration blocked the enhancement of ascorbate biosynthesis brought about by barbituric acid or 3-MC.

2. Microsome- and Membrane-Bound Enzymes: In a sustained series of penetrating researches, Warburg 1948*a, b* discovered that atmospheric O_2 consumed by respiring cells does not react directly with cell metabolites. Rather, O_2 combines with and oxidizes a divalent iron complex, which in turn delivers oxygen to the cell substrates. Warburg 1948*a, b* discovered the light-reversible carbon monoxide inhibition of respiration in yeast. This observation provided evidence for the cytochrome nature of the enzymes of respiration that had been found out by Keilin 1925.

Mueller and Miller 1949 discovered that insoluble particulate fractions of rat liver homogenates in the presence of O_2 and NADPH catalyzed the reductive cleavage (reductase) of the azo bridge of the strong hepatic carcinogen 4-dimethylaminoazobenzene (DAB) to yield monophenylamines. Mueller and Miller 1953 also described the enzymatic oxidative demethylation (N-demethylase) in liver of N-monomethyl azo dyes related to DAB.

Brodie et al. 1955 discovered a common enzyme denominator in the metabolism of foreign compounds. The 'Brodie enzymes" are localized in and bound to hepatic microsomes; they are not present in cytosols; they have a strict activity requirement for molecular O_2 and NADPH. Brodie et al. 1955 found that many metabolic activities are brought about by these microsomal enzymes, including dealkylation, deamination, ether cleavage, hydroxylation, and others. One of the striking properties of the microsomal enzyme system is the wide variety of aromatic compounds it can hydroxylate and, consequently, detoxify. The extent of hydroxylation is related to polarity of the substrate; an increase of polarity in an aromatic compound inhibits attack by the microsomal system. Udenfriend et al. 1954 found that aromatic hydroxylation can be accomplished nonenzymatically by the systems [$H_2O_2 + Fe^{2+}$] and [ascorbic acid $+ O_2 + Fe^{2+}$].

Mason 1957 studied a group of biological oxidation reactions in which atmospheric O_2 was incorporated into the substrate instead of serving as a terminal electron acceptor. The hydroxylation of various aromatic compounds by the liver and the hydroxylation of steroids constitute a subgroup of cellular oxidations with common features: *i*, association with microsomes, *ii*, noninhibition by cyanide, and *iii*, dependence on atmospheric O_2 and NADPH. Mason 1957 introduced the term mixed function oxidases for enzymes catalyzing this type of hydroxylation; it was postulated that one atom of O_2 was incorporated into the organic molecule while the second atom was reduced to form water.

Estabrook, Cooper, and Rosenthal 1963 identified the oxygen-activating enzyme for hydroxylation (at position C_{21}) of 17-hydroxyprogesterone; the reaction, carried out by microsomes of bovine adrenal cortex, is inhibited by CO and the inhibition is reversed by light. Spectrophotometry revealed the appearance of an absorption band (λ_{max}, 450 mμ) when CO was added to adrenal microsomes that had been reduced by NADPH. The newly formed absorption band, designated P-450, is a cytochrome oxidase located on the smooth endoplasmic reticulum, an anatomical structure, devoid of microsomes, which forms a branching tubular network in the cytoplasm.

Conney and Klutch 1963 found that treatment of rats with phenobarbital for 4 days stimulated the activity in liver microsomes of enzyme systems that hydroxylate testosterone and 4-androstene-3,17-dione; the androgen system requires NADPH and molecular O_2 for its activity. Phenobarbital stimulates the synthesis of cytochrome P-450 and causes a striking increase in smooth endoplasmic reticulum membranes.

Haugen, Coon, and Nebert 1976 described the genetic control of multiple forms of induction of cytochrome oxidases in mouse liver. The administration of aromatic compounds such as β-naphthoflavone or 3-MC causes the induction of many different hepatic microsomal monoxygenase activities together with the appearance of a distinct cytochrome, P-448, in genetically responsive but not in nonresponsive mouse strains. However, the administration of 2,3,7,8-tetrachlorodibenzo-*p*-dioxin induces these enzyme activities and cytochrome P-448 formation to the same extent in both responsive and nonresponsive inbred strains of mice. In contrast, phenobarbital induces in both responsive and nonresponsive strains a different profile of enzyme activities and the appearance of cytochrome P-450 rather than cytochrome P-448.

3. Menadione Reductase: Martius and Märki 1957 isolated in highly purified form from beef liver a soluble diaphorase that catalyzes the oxidation of NADH and NADPH by various redox dyes and quinones. Menadione reductase (EC 1.6.99.2) reacts strongly with menadione (2-methyl-1,4-naphthoquinone) and

weakly with vitamin K_1. The enzyme is a flavoprotein characterized by an efficient and specific inhibition by dicumarol (Märki and Martius 1960).

Among the striking properties (Ernster, Ljunggren, and Danielson 1960) of menadione reductase are these, *i*, it reacts with many electron acceptors including coenzyme Q and 2,6-dichlorophenolindophenol; *ii*, it is found both in liver cytosol and in microsomal membranes; *iii*, it is inhibited by flavin antagonists including atebrin, chlorpromazine, and thyroxin; and *iv*, dicumarol is the most potent inhibitor; the enzyme is inhibited (50%) in 10^{-8} M dicumarol.

It was a novel finding that many foreign substances of an organic nature induce the formation of this soluble enzyme, menadione reductase, in liver, lung, fat, mammary cancer, and other tissues (Williams-Ashman and Huggins 1961; Huggins and Fukunishi 1964). The assay (method 6.3) of MR in soluble extracts of tissues is simple, rapid, and reproducible; the reaction follows zero-order kinetics.

Williams-Ashman and Huggins 1961 observed that 3 days after a single feeding of 20 mg of 7,12-DMBA to S-D female rats, MR was increased twofold in aqueous extracts of mammary gland and perirenal fat.

The induction of menadione reductase in liver was studied following a single feeding of aromatic hydrocarbons. All of the compounds induced the formation of the enzyme. The most potent inducer was Sudan III, followed by 3-MC, 7,12-DMBA, BA, and 7,8,12-TMBA (table 10.1).

Table 10.1   Induction of Hepatic Menadione Reductase by Aromatic Compounds

		Menadione reductase	
Compound	Protein mg/100 mg	units/100 mg	units/1 mg protein
None (controls)	12.4 ± 0.6	2.6 ± 0.3	0.21
7,8,12-TMBA	9.2 ± 0.5	6.5 ± 2.0	0.70
BA	10.4 ± 1.3	7.9 ± 1.8	0.76
7,12-DMBA	9.4 ± 0.3	10.7 ± 1.5	1.14
3-MC	10.8 ± 0.4	13.0 ± 1.5	1.20
Sudan III	13.2 ± 0.2	18.9 ± 1.2	1.44

NOTE: 10 mg of aromatic compound dissolved in 2 ml of sesame oil was fed by gastric instillation to L-E rats, age 49 days; controls were fed 2 ml of sesame oil. Liver was harvested at age 50 days. Each group consisted of 4 rats; two samples from each animal were assayed by method 6.3. Means with standard deviation ± are given.

Prevention of 7,12-DMBA-Produced Adrenal Apoplexy

In addition to inducing cancer in a spectacular way, 7,12-DMBA causes massive hormone-dependent necrosis of a wide stratum in the middle of the adrenal gland of rat under stated conditions (p. 130). It has been found that adrenocorticolysis of this special sort with adrenal apoplexy can be prevented by any of a number of aromatic compounds provided the protector is given prior to 7,12-DMBA. Those compounds that induced protection against selective adrenal destruction also protected, to a lesser or greater extent, against hydrocarbon-induced malignant disease. The assay (method 10.1) of compounds effective in the prevention of 7,12-DMBA-produced adrenal necrosis is a simple and rapid screening to identify and evaluate the potency of those substances which lessen the incidence of leukemia and mammary cancer.

Method 10.1: Protection of Adrenal Cortex against 7,12-DMBA

In studying adrenal protection (Huggins and Pataki 1965) there were in each group 5 normal female S-D rats, age 46–49 days, weighing 140–160 g. On day -1, the animals were fed by gastric instillation a single dose of compound to be evaluated as a protector dissolved in sesame oil, 2 ml. In investigating the possible protective value of a compound, a preliminary series of dose levels (e.g., 100 mg, 10 mg, 1 mg) was given. On day 0, 1 ml of a lipid emulsion containing 5 mg of 7,12-DMBA was injected in a caudal vein. On day 3 adrenals were harvested and weighed, and the content of hemoglobin in the right adrenal was measured.

Dao and Tanaka 1963a found that feeding 30 mg of 3-MC on each of two successive days before feeding 30 mg of 7,12-DMBA inhibited completely the necrosis-inducing action of 7,12-DMBA; the adrenal cortex of rats treated with 3-MC prior to 7,12-DMBA did not suffer injury.

Huggins and Fukunishi 1964 investigated the time relationship of protector to challenger in S-D female rats, age 50 days. The protector was 2 mg of 3-MC; the challenger was 5 mg of 7,12-DMBA. Protector and challenger were given by intravenous injection. The biological indicator was the presence or absence of gross hemorrhage in the adrenal glands 72 hr after administration of the challenging dose of 7,12-DMBA. Adrenal apoplexy is a dramatic phenomenon clearly evident to the unaided eye.

Massive adrenal necrosis results when protector and challenger are injected together. Intravenous injection of a single solution containing both 7,12-DMBA, 5 mg, *plus* 3-MC, 2–10 mg, invariably led to adrenal apoplexy in every animal. The inducer of protection must be injected before the challenger in order to be effective. The injection of a small dose of 3-MC (2 mg) exerted the following influence: *i*, the time of protection (*t*) was 2 hr $< t <$ 3 hr; *ii*, protection lasted only 2 days; *iii*, a small dose of ethionine (25 mg) blocked the induction of protection by 3-MC; *iv*, this single dose of ethionine (25 mg) blocked protection when the amino acid was given as late as 2 hr after 3-MC. The last item is especially noteworthy since ethionine blocked protection a few minutes before the induction of drug-metabolizing enzymes was established. Administration of ethionine 4 hr after 3-MC had no effect on the protective process since the protective enzymes already had been synthesized.

Thirteen aromatic compounds were assayed for their ability to protect the adrenal cortex from destruction by 7,12-DMBA; 6 of the compounds were azo dyes and 7 compounds were polycyclic aromatic hydrocarbons. The azo dyes (table 10.2) were more potent in establishing protection and the most efficacious inducer of protection was Sudan III (compound I).

Table 10.2   Aromatic Compounds Inducing Adrenal Protection

No.	Compound	Minimum protective dose, mg
	1. Azo Dyes	
I	1-(*p*-Phenylazo-phenylazo)-2-naphthol	0.01
II	1-(*p*-Phenylazo-phenylazo)-1-naphthalene	0.05
III	1-(*o*-Tolylazo-*o*-tolylazo)-2-naphthol	0.05
IV	1,2′-Azonaphthalene	0.1
V	1-(1-Naphthylazo)-2-naphthol	0.1
VI	1,1′-Azonaphthalene	0.1
	2. Polycyclic Hydrocarbons	
VII	3-Methylcholanthrene	0.25
VIII	Benzo[*a*]pyrene	0.5
IX	Benz[*a*]anthracene	1.0
X	7,12-Diethylbenz[*a*]anthracene	1.0
XI	Diels hydrocarbon	1.0
XII	Cyclopentenophenanthrene	2.0
XIII	7,12-Dimethylbenz[*a*]anthracene	2.0

NOTE: On day -1, S-D female rats, age 49 days, were fed a single dose of compound dissolved in 2 ml of sesame oil. On day 0, 7,12-DMBA, 5 mg, was injected intravenously. On day 3, the adrenals were harvested. Minimum protective dose prevents adrenal apoplexy in all members of a group of 5–8 rats.

Microsome-Bound Drug-Metabolizing Enzymes

The major metabolites of the potent carcinogen benzo[a]pyrene are monohydroxy derivatives which are weakly active or inactive as carcinogens; subsequently noncarcinogenic quinones and epoxides are formed. Conney, Miller, and Miller 1957 discovered the enzymatic hydroxylation of BP by fortified rat liver homogenates. Benzpyrene hydroxylase is localized in the microsomes and is not present in hepatic cytosols; it requires NADPH and molecular O_2 for activity. Fluorescence of BP metabolites is the basis of the enzyme assay.

The intraperitoneal injection of BP into weanling rats caused a rapid increase in hepatic benzpyrene hydroxylase to $\sim$ 5 to 10 times the control value within 24 hr. The carcinogens DBA and 3-MC are fully as active as BP itself in the induction of hepatic benzpyrene hydroxylase, whereas 7,12-DMBA was only one-third as active in this regard. The response to benzo[a]pyrene is prevented by the administration of ethionine; the effect of ethionine is nullified by the simultaneous administration of methionine.

Wattenberg, Leong, and Strand 1962 found that the oral administration of benz[a]anthracene caused a profound increase in BP-hydroxylase activity in liver and throughout the entire gastrointestinal tract.

The induction of BP-hydroxylase in liver by 3-MC is inhibited by puromycin or actinomycin D; therefore, the changes in the hydroxylase levels are dependent on protein and RNA synthesis (Gelboin and Blackburn 1964).

Wattenberg and Leong 1965 found that phenothiazine and several of its derivatives are potent inducers of BP-hydroxylase activity. These phenothiazines also protected rats against adrenal necrosis following a massive oral dose of 7,12-DMBA.

Azo Dye-Induced Prevention of Mammary Cancer

It is possible to prevent cancer of the breast in many rats but, as yet, not in every animal (Huggins, Grand, and Fukunishi 1964). The basis of our experiment is that a single feeding of 20 mg of 7,12-DMBA will induce mammary carcinoma in more than 95% of S-D rats at risk (p. 73). In preliminary experiments a compound to be evaluated as an inducer of protection against breast cancer was chosen for its ability to protect the adrenal cortex against massive hemorrhage caused by 7,12-DMBA and for its efficiency in the induction of hepatic menadione in rat. In our experiments the most efficient compound in these regards was 1-(p-phenylazo-phenylazo)-2-naphthol (Sudan III).

Young adult S-D female rats were fed Sudan III, 1 mg or 10 mg, dissolved in 2 ml of sesame oil at −48 hr and again at −24 hr; at 0 hr every rat was fed a single dose of 20 mg of 7,12-DMBA (∼ 130 mg/kg). The resulting incidence of mammary cancer (table 10.3) was Sudan III, 1 mg, 82%; Sudan III, 10 mg, 55%; and controls 100%.

Table 10.3   Sudan III-Induced Prevention of Mammary Carcinoma in Female Rats Fed a Carcinogenic Dose of 7,12-DMBA

Azo dye	Dose (mg)	Number of rats at risk	Mammary cancer detection	
			Number of rats	Range (days)
Sudan III	1	17	14 (82%)	53.5 ± 18
Sudan III	10	11	6 (55%)	63.5 ± 16
None (controls)	—	11	11 (100%)	37.4 ± 14

NOTE: S-D female rats were fed Sudan III, 1 mg or 10 mg, in 2 ml of sesame oil by gastric instillation at −48 hr and again at −24 hr; controls were fed 2 ml of sesame oil. At age 50 days every rat was given a single feeding of 20 mg of 7,12-DMBA in 2ml of sesame oil. Means with standard deviation ± are given.

Azo Dye-Induced Prevention of Hydrocarbon-Induced Leukemia

Proposition 13: Prevention of Leukemia

Small quantities (1 to 10 mg) of 1-(p-phenylazo-phenylazo)-2-naphthol fed by gastric instillation to Long-Evans female rats are highly effective in preventing hydrocarbon-induced leukemia when a feeding of azo dye is given prior to every dose of a leukemogenic set of intravenous injections of 7,8,12-trimethylbenz[a]anthracene.

Beginning at age 50 days, L-E male rats were given a series of 4 intravenous injections of 7,8,12-TMBA, 35 mg/kg, at biweekly intervals. Sudan III, 1 mg or 10 mg in 2 ml of sesame oil, was fed by gastric instillation at 48 hr and again at 24 hr before each injection (Huggins, Ueda, and Russo 1978). The resulting incidence of leukemia (table 10.4) was Sudan III, 1 mg, 6%; Sudan III, 10 mg, no rat; and controls 92%.

Table 10.4   Sudan III-Induced Prevention of Leukemia in Rats Given
                                a Leukemogenic Series of Injections of 7,8,12-TMBA

Azo dye	Dose (mg)	at risk Number of rats	Leukemia detection	
			Number of rats	Range (days)
Sudan III	1	16	1 (6%)	83
Sudan III	10	14	0	—
None (controls)	—	13	12 (92%)	60.1 ± 15

NOTE: Beginning at age 50 days, L-E male rats were given a series of 4 intravenous injections of 7,8,12-TMBA, 35 mg/kg, at biweekly intervals. Sudan III, 1 mg or 10 mg, dissolved in 2 ml of sesame oil was fed by gastric instillation at −48 hr and again at −24 hr before each injection. Controls were fed 2 ml of sesame oil. Mean with standard deviation ± is given.

Failure of Sudan III to Elicit Tumors

In the experiments of Fischer 1906, a saturated solution of Scarlet Red in olive oil, designated Scharlachöl, was assayed for carcinogenicity in the ears of rabbits by subcutaneous injection or by repeated skin paintings. The rabbits were observed for many months but cancer failed to arise in the animals.

In the experiments of Huggins, Ueda, and Russo 1978, Sudan III was tested for carcinogenicity in L-E rats. *i.* A solution of Sudan III, 0.5% w/v, in sesame oil was prepared; 0.5 ml of the solution was injected in thigh muscle of both legs of 8 rats age 27 days; the animals were observed for 9 months. At necropsy on day 276 a residual depot of red, dye-colored oil was found at every injection site but sarcomas were not present. *ii.* A solution of Sudan III, 0.1% w/v, in sesame oil was prepared. A group of 16 female rats was fed by gastric instillation, 1 ml of the solution 5 times each week for 26 weeks. Ten animals survived for 40 weeks. At necropsy no tumors were observed in the liver or elsewhere.

Preservation of Life of Rats Given a Massive Dose of 7,12-DMBA

Huggins, Ford et al. 1964 found out that in the rat a small amount of 3-MC given before a massive, highly toxic dose of 7,12-DMBA induced a physiologic state that protected the recipient from the otherwise lethal amount so that life was preserved.

It will be recalled that LD_{50} for a single intravenous injection of 7,12-DMBA in rats is $\sim$54–58 mg/kg. An injection of 7,12-DMBA, 133 mg/kg, caused the death of 20 consecutive rats, age 46 days, in 16–21 hr. There was a remarkable uniformity in their clinical status. There were no pronounced changes in behavior in the early hours after the injection of 7,12-DMBA. The animals had alternating short periods of activity and sleep, a pattern similar to that of untreated rats in a well-illuminated room. The injected rats ate little or no food but drank much water. After 2–5 hr ears, paws, and tail become red from vaso-dilatation, and this persisted until death. Abruptly at 8.0–9.5 hr there was a copious evacuation of watery stool containing much mucous; diarrhea continued until death. At 10 hr the animals looked sick and the fur was untidy; they remained crouched, somnolent, and inactive (fig. 10.1). The eyes were watery and the animals were cold to the touch. There was an agonal convulsion followed in a few minutes by death at 16–21 hr.

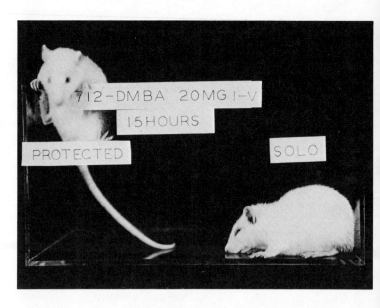

Fig. 10.1. Two rats, age 46 days, were injected with 20 mg of 7,12-DMBA (~130 mg/kg) at 0 hr; the photograph was taken 15 hr later. One rat (*left*) which had been injected with 2 mg of 3-MC 24 hr prior to 7,12-DMBA is active; its sister (*right*), which had not received 3-MC, is moribund. The injections were intravenous.

All rats injected with 3-MC, 2 mg (~ 13 mg/kg) on day −1, survived injection of 7,12-DMBA, 20 mg, on day 0. Their re-action was very different from that of rats receiving 20 mg of 7,12-DMBA without prior injection of 3-MC. There was an initial loss of weight but recovery was evident on day 2. There was no diarrhea or convulsions. There were no obvious signs that the animals had been given a dose of 7,12-DMBA, which was overwhelming in the absence of protection established in advance.

In the experiments of Huggins, Ueda, and Russo 1978, a group of 16 female L-E rats, age 38 days, was given a single intravenous injection of 7,12-DMBA, 75 mg/kg; every animal succumbed in 1–3 days. An identical group of female rats was given a single feeding of 0.1 mg of Sudan III dissolved in 1 ml of sesame oil by gastric instillation 24 hr prior to an intravenous injection of 7,12-DMBA; there were no deaths. The procedure (Sudan III feeding and subsequent 7,12-DMBA injection) was repeated thrice at intervals of 21 days. There were no deaths but leukemia developed in 8 of 16 rats; leukemia was detected in 60–74 days, mean 63.5 ± 6.5 days.

Lymphomas and Ovarian Tumors
Elicited by 7,12-DMBA in Mouse

The induction of cancer by hydrocarbons is determined by a conjunction of two components, the genetic constitution and the carcinogen; these factors, equal in significance, are crucial in importance. Cancer arises when a potent carcinogen alters a susceptible genetic code in a specific way. The dual factors are clearly evident in the genesis of malignant tumors in mouse. Consider, for example, 3-methylcholanthrene—this carcinogen, acting in pure-line strains of mice, causes the incidence of leukemias and lymphomas as follows: dba strain 98%, C3H 5%, C albino 0 (Morton and Mider 1941).

In a group of susceptible animals carcinogens accelerate the time of appearance and augment the incidence of cancers that might appear spontaneously in their absence, albeit more slowly and in lower percentage. Carcinogens do not produce grotesque and unnatural growths that would not form spontaneously in their absence.

In mice of certain strains, polycyclic aromatic hydrocarbons preferentially elicit lymphomas in high yield. The methods of induction of these neoplasms are simple. In mouse 7,12-DMBA is the most effective of the carcinogenic hydrocarbons. The polycyclic aromatic hydrocarbons have a special attribute in the mouse; 7,12-DMBA and 3-MC elicit ovarian tumors in mouse in high yield. These aromatics do not produce tumors of the ovary in rat.

The predominant hematopoietic neoplasms elicited by the aromatics in mouse are lymphosarcoma of the thymus and lymphocytic leukemia; less common are erythroleukemia and myelocytic leukemia. The hydrocarbon-induced neoplasms of the lymphatic system are especially useful for investigative purposes for three reasons: *i*, whereas lymphatic leukemia is elicited in mouse in high yield, this sort of leukemia seldom occurs in rat; *ii*, in common with lymphomas of man, neoplasms of the lymphatic system are hormone-responsive and frequently regress in a dramatic way (some are cured) following the administration of glucocorticoids; *iii*, many lymphomas of mouse regress after the injection of guinea pig serum or *L*-asparaginase (Kidd 1953).

Hydrocarbon-Induced Neoplasms in Inbred Mice

Lymphomas Induced by 3-MC. In 1909 Little developed a strain of mice with light brown fur by recombination of coat-color genes (see Little 1958). Brother × sister matings were started at once and one of the homogeneous strains (dba) survived and has been perpetuated; this study was the origin of pure-line strains of mice in America.

The induction of lymphomas by the surgeons Morton and Mider (1938) initiated a vast field of cancer research. The experimental animals were virgin female dba mice. Commencing at age 4–6 weeks, the skin of the mice was painted, using a camel's hair brush, at semiweekly intervals with a solution containing 0.5% 3-MC in benzene; the locus of application of the hydrocarbon was changed with each painting; 9 sites in all were used. On day 69 the first tumor was detected; it was a lymphosarcoma in the inguinal region with generalized lymphadenopathy (Morton and Mider 1938).

Morton and Mider 1941 confirmed and extended their earlier observations in which mice of dba strain were painted with 3-MC. The incidence of lymphomas was more than 98%. These neoplasms were detected rather rapidly: males at 86.1 ± 13 days and females at 90 ± 11 days. Age and sex of the recipients had little effect on the development of lymphomas but genetic constitution had a profound influence.

In the experiments of Morton and Mider 1941 three sorts of lymphoma were observed: first and most frequent generalized lymphomatosis with great enlargement of liver, spleen, and lymph nodes (75% of mice); second, solitary lymphosarcoma of thymus (21% of mice) without involvement of lymph nodes, liver, or spleen; and, third, reticuloendotheliosis (< 5%).

In addition, Morton and Mider 1941 painted a group of dba mice at semiweekly intervals with a solution of 0.5% benzo[*a*]-pyrene in benzene; 62% of the mice developed leukosis. A control group of dba mice was painted with benzene alone and observed for 1.5 years; 23% of the mice developed generalized lymphomatosis.

Lymphomas Induced by 7,12-DMBA. In the experiments of Law 1941, mice of the dba strain were painted at semiweekly intervals with a solution containing 0.5% 7,12-DMBA in benzene. Generalized lymphomatosis (lymphatic leukemia) developed in 85% of the mice; the mean latent period was 107.6 days. Among control mice untreated with hydrocarbon the incidence of lymphoma was 30%. From a similar experiment Law and Lewisohn 1940 concluded: "Given the hereditary predisposition to tumor formation, the application of certain carcinogens will hasten the appearance and in some instances increase the incidence of the tumor."

Haran-Ghera, Kotler, and Meshorer 1967 studied the SJL/J strain of mice in which spontaneous reticulum cell neoplasms appeared in 70%–80% of intact mice at a mean age of 380 days. Multiple feedings of a solution of 7,12-DMBA (1 mg per feeding) by gastric tube induced lymphatic leukemia in 74% of the mice at an average latent period of 174 days. The animals developed the syndrome of an enlarged thymus with involvement of lymph nodes, liver, and spleen. Few reticulum cell sarcomas (7 to 15%) developed in the mice. It was of interest that lymphatic leukemia developed in high yield in this strain of thymectomized mice.

Ovarian Tumors and Mammary Carcinoma Elicited by Carcinogens. It is now well established that mammary cancer and ovarian granulosa-cell tumors can be induced separately or together by means of chemical carcinogens in mice of various strains free from the milk factor. Biancifiori, Bonser, and Cashera 1961 found that in regard to mammary cancer 7,12-DMBA and 3-MC are equivalent in potency, whereas in the production of ovarian tumors 7,12-DMBA is the more potent carcinogen. All of the ovarian tumors in their experiments were of granulosa-cell type.

Howell, Marchant, and Orr 1954 were the first to elicit ovarian tumors with polycyclic aromatic hydrocarbons. Young virgin female mice of a purebred line (IF strain) and their F_1 hybrids were studied; drops of a solution (olive oil) containing 0.5% 7,12-DMBA were applied to the skin at biweekly intervals. The incidence of neoplasms was 74% with mammary cancer and 60% with ovarian tumors. The earliest ovarian tumor was detected 4 months after the first skin painting; all of the tumors of the ovary appeared to originate in granulosa cells. Extending the foregoing experiments, Marchant 1957 applied 7,12-DMBA to the skin of mice of several purebred lines. The incidence of ovarian tumors in the various strains was: IF strain 40%–70%, A strain 0, and C3H strain 0.

Hydrocarbon-Induced Neoplasms in Noninbred Mice

CF-1 mice are albinos that have been randomly bred among themselves for scores of generations. They constitute a stock especially advantageous for leukemia research (Uematsu and Huggins 1968, 1969), for several reasons. CF-1 mice have remained free from epidemics of infectious diseases for more than a decade. They are also commercially available from several dealers at low cost; they breed rapidly and nurture large litters and so a big colony can be assembled quickly. Leukemia and ovarian tumors occur spontaneously in low incidence but are elicited in 2–3 months in profusion by simple methods; mammary cancer is uncommon. The induced leukemias of CF-1 mice are readily transplanted subcutaneously to newborn mice of the same stock.

Leukemia in the mouse manifests itself in 4 syndromes: *i*, dyspnea, dilated jugular veins, and exophthalmos caused by lymphosarcoma of the thymus; mice with this syndrome usually succumb within 5 days; *ii*, prominent superficial lymph nodes, usually bilateral, in cervical, axillary, and inguinal lymph nodes; the lymph nodes of normal mice are not palpable; *iii*, enlarged abdomen due to hepatomegaly and splenomegaly; and *iv*, persistent loss of weight over a period of 5 days or longer.

The venous blood of mice with thymic leukemia (syndrome i) is characterized by values of hemoglobin and hematocrit similar to those of normal controls. Mice with syndromes ii–iv are anemic.

There were 15 mice with spontaneous tumors in a control group of 103 untreated virgin female CF-1 mice observed for 17 months (Uematsu and Huggins 1968). The tumors were leukemia 7, mammary cancer 4, ovarian 1, pulmonary 1, cutaneous 1, and soft tissue sarcoma 1.

Toxicity of 7,12-DMBA and 7,8,12-TMBA

The dosage of hydrocarbons that caused the death of half of a group of rodents (LD_{50}) in 21 days was determined by the probit method of Gaddum (see Burn, Finney, and Goodwin 1950) after a single intravenous injection of emulsions of polycyclic aromatic hydrocarbons in CF-1 mouse and L-E rat, age 42–54 days. Remarkable differences between these species were found (table 11.1). A single pulse-injection of 7,12-DMBA is not toxic for mouse but very toxic for rat; 7,8,12-TMBA is highly toxic for mouse but relatively nontoxic for rat.

Method 11.1: Induction of Leukemia in Mouse

CF-1 female mice were purchased from a dealer (Charles River Breeding Laboratories, Inc., Wilmington, Mass.) and housed

Table 11.1   Differential Toxicity in Rat and Mouse of Polycyclic
                             Aromatic Hydrocarbons Given by Intravenous Injection

	LD_{50}	
	Rat	Mouse
Hydrocarbon		mg/kg
BA	>200	>200
7,12-DMBA	40	>200
7,8,12-TMBA	90	50

NOTE: Female L-E rats and CF-1 mice, age 42–53 days, were given a
single pulse-injection of hydrocarbon and observed for 21 days. There
were 8 animals in each set at each dose level.

in plastic boxes (8/cage) in air-conditioned rooms at $25° \pm 1°$.
The animals were fed a commercial ration (Rockland Mouse/
Rat Diet, Teklad, Inc., Monmouth, Ill.) and given tap water
ad libitum.

The carcinogen 7,12-DMBA, m.p. 122°–123° (Eastman
Kodak Co., Rochester, N.Y.), was refined by Florisil
chromatography and recrystallized from acetone-ethanol.
Gastric Instillation:

For gastric instillation a solution (sesame oil) of purified
7,12-DMBA, 1% w/v, was prepared by heating the mixture
for 30 min at 100°C. Gastric tubes were made from flexible
polyethylene tubing (diameter 2 mm); any sharp ends of the
tubing were blunted by heating in the flame of a match.

A mouse was anesthetized with ether and fed by tube a dose
of 2.5 mg 7,12-DMBA dissolved in 0.25 ml of oil; 4 similar
feedings were given at biweekly intervals.
Intravenous Injection:

For intravenous injection a lipid emulsion containing 7,12-
DMBA, 0.5% w/w, was prepared by the method of Schurr
(see appendix 2). A mouse holder was made from a plastic
cylinder, capped at both ends, in which holes are bored;
the dimensions of the cylinder were length 9 cm and diameter
2.5 cm. The mouse was inserted in the holder allowing the
tail to protrude from a hole in one of the caps. The tail was
immersed briefly in warm water (43°C) and the emulsion was
injected in a dilated caudal vein; a dose of 1.0 mg 7,12-DMBA
was repeated at biweekly intervals.

Induction of Leukemia by   A set of 8 intravenous injections of 7,12-DMBA (40–50 mg/
Intravenous Injection of   kg) was administered to a series of 32 female mice of CF-1
7,12-DMBA in Mouse   strain: each dose of 7,12-DMBA was 1 mg and the injections

were given at biweekly intervals starting at age 8 weeks. Two mice (6%) succumbed prematurely. In 30 effective mice the incidence of neoplasms was leukemia in 29 mice (97%), cancer of the ovary in 15 (50%), and mammary cancer in 6 (20%). Leukemia was observed at 66–115 days (mean 95.5 ± 15).

Proposition 14:
Induction of Leukemia
in CF-1 Mouse

Leukemia is elicited in more than 90% of heterozygous female mice of CF-1 strain given a set of 8 intravenous injections of 7,12-dimethylbenz[a]anthracene at biweekly intervals starting in the age period, 4 to 8 weeks. Each dose of 7,12-DMBA is 1 mg.

**Induction of Leukemia by
Feeding 7,12-DMBA
in Mouse**

In the experiments of Huggins and Uematsu 1976, 49 female mice, age 6–7 weeks, were given 4 feedings of 7,12-DMBA at biweekly intervals. Each feeding comprised 2.5 mg of 7,12-DMBA dissolved in 0.25 ml of sesame oil. The mouse was anesthetized briefly for ease of gastric instillation.

Eight mice died of aplastic anemia; 41 mice, designated effective, survived 50+ days and malignant neoplasms were found in 39 of them (table 11.2): 30 had leukemia, 24 had ovarian tumors, and 2 had mammary carcinoma. Some mice had multiple tumors. Leukemias detected in 73% of the effective mice were observed in 71–164 days (mean 112 ± 24 days). The mammary cancers were squamous carcinomas; ovarian tumors were of granulosa-cell or luteoma type.

Table 11.2

Neoplasms in CF-1 Mice Elicited by Multiple Feedings of 7,12-DMBA

No. of mice			Type of neoplasm		
Original	Effective	Developing neoplasms	Leukemia	Ovary	Mammary cancer
a. 7,12-DMBA Feedings					
49	41	39	30	24	4
b. Controls					
103	103	8	7	1	0

NOTE: Four feedings of 2.5 mg of 7,12-DMBA were given at biweekly intervals to female CF-1 mice; the first dose was fed at age 50 days. Controls were untreated.

Ovarian tumors (Uematsu and Huggins 1969) were round or oval and yellow in color and had dilated blood vessels and hemorrhagic spots. Frequently they grew to a size greater than

1 cm in diameter and in mice with these large tumors the contralateral ovary was small and atrophic. Uematsu and Huggins 1968 transplanted ovaries of untreated control mice to a subcutaneous pocket in the ears; 2 of 6 normal mice with transplants of this sort observed for 17 months developed granulosa-cell tumors in the grafted ovaries.

Inoculation of Newborn Mice with Leukemic Blood

At age 1 day, CF-1 infants were inoculated subcutaneously with 0.05–0.1 ml leukemic blood. There were 236 infants that survived 14+ days (table 11.3); either lymphatic leukemia or lymphosarcoma or both neoplasms occurred in 107 of the infants (Huggins and Uematsu 1976). Leukemia was detected in the infant mice 10–56 days after the inoculation; the mean time of detection was 21.4 ± 11 days.

Table 11.3

Lymphosarcoma and Leukemia Following Inoculation of Whole Blood from Leukemic Mice into Newborn

Number of Donors	56
Number of Newborn Recipients	274
Effective Recipients	236
Total Number of Takes	107
Lymphosarcoma Alone	43
Leukemia Alone	15
Lymphosarcoma and Leukemia	49

NOTE: Donors and recipients were CF-1 mice.

Influence of Adrenalectomy and Glucocorticoids on Lymphomas

Murphy and Sturm 1943 found that adrenalectomy enhanced the growth of transplanted lymphosarcoma in rat. With respect to adrenalectomy the animals were more susceptible to inoculated leukemia, the lymphomas grew more rapidly, and the adrenalectomized rats survived a shorter time than control mates.

Dougherty and White 1943 found that the administration of corticotrophin (ACTH) to intact normal mouse causes a profound diminution in size of all lymph nodes, thymus, and the entire lymphatic apparatus. Heilman and Kendall 1944 administered large amounts of cortisone to mice bearing a transplanted lymphosarcoma and stated: "Although dramatic and apparently complete cures are produced, they are only temporary in a majority of animals. . . . After an interval of a few days or weeks the tumors usually recur and this time they are completely refractory."

Pearson et al. 1949 found that corticotrophin or cortisone caused dramatic if temporary regression in certain cases of human lymphatic leukemia and Hodgkin's disease.

L-asparaginase-Induced Regression of Lymphomas

Kidd 1953 found that in mouse transplanted lymphomas of two kinds regularly regressed following repeated intraperitoneal injections of normal guinea pig serum; the animals remained healthy. Sera of horse and rabbit failed to cause a regression. Lymphomas of untreated control mice grew rapidly and killed their hosts in 20–30 days. Two transplanted mammary cancers grew unimpeded in mice injected with guinea pig serum.

Broome 1963 found that the properties of L-asparaginase (asp) were indistinguishable from the antilymphoma agent of guinea pig serum. Ten new mouse lymphomas were found to be sensitive to the inhibitory effects of asp. The enzyme is active only when given to animals in vivo; it had no effect on lymphoma cells in vitro. When 1–2 ml of guinea pig serum was injected intraperitoneally in mice bearing lymphomas, complete suppression of the tumor occurred in some animals. If asp is in fact the tumor-inhibiting factor in guinea pig serum, its inhibitory activity on tumor cells of sensitive lines is very much more powerful than that produced by other enzymes that have been tested, including ribonuclease and xanthine oxidase.

Capizzi et al. 1969 reported a series of 6 clinical patients with acute lymphocytic leukemia treated with L-asparaginase. All patients experienced dramatic objective improvement in their disease in 3–4 days and 4 patients had complete remissions.

Glucocorticoid-Induced Regression of Transplanted Leukemia and Lymphosarcoma

A suspension of dexamethasone in saline was tested for toxicity in CF-1 mice, age 50 days; at 21 days the LD_{50} for intraperitoneal injection was 140 mg/kg. A single feeding of dexamethasone, 220 mg/kg, caused no mortality.

In the experiments of Huggins and Uematsu 1976 newborn mice were inoculated subcutaneously with 0.05 ml of leukemic whole blood obtained by cardiac puncture from CF-1 mice in the terminal stages of leukemia; 29 mice developed lymphosarcoma at the site of inoculation. The animals were tube-fed large doses of corticosteroids on 1–4 occasions.

In 1 mouse there was no response to the administration of corticosteroids. In 28 mice there was a dramatic regression of the lymphosarcomas. In the favorable cases the tumor was less than half its original size within 24 hr after the first feeding of cortisone or dexamethasone. In 16 mice (table 11.3) the lymphosarcoma disappeared but recurred within 7 days after its disappearance. In 4 mice there was complete regression without recurrence in 61–82 days.

In summary, a set of tube-feedings of 7,12-DMBA elicited in CF-1 mice lymphatic leukemias in high yield. CF-1 mice with the thymic type of lymphoma died within 5 days after dyspnea was detected. The inoculation of whole blood of mice with lymphatic leukemia into allogeneic newborn gave rise to local lymphosarcoma at the injection site. The transplanted lymphosarcomas are advantageous for investigation for several reasons: *i*, their hosts survived for several weeks after the local neoplasm was detected; *ii*, growth or regression of the lymphosarcoma is easily measured; and *iii*, many of the lymphosarcomas regress when glucocorticoids are fed. In 14% of mice there was no recurrence of lymphosarcoma in 2.5 months after treatment with glucocorticoids.

Immunologic Inhibition of the Adenohypophysis

Pierpaoli and Haran-Ghera 1975 observed many congenital endocrine derangements in SJL/J mice, a strain characterized by a high incidence of spontaneous reticulum-cell sarcomas. This observation led to an investigation of the effect of antiadenohypophysis (anti-AH) serum on mice subjected to different leukemia-producing agents, namely, *i*, total body x-irradiation, or *ii*, gastric instillation of 1 mg 7,12-DMBA at weekly intervals for 5 doses. The pituitary antibodies were obtained from sheep serum. At intervals, intraperitoneal inoculation with anti-AH serum was carried out during and after exposure to the carcinogenic agents. It was found that anti-AH antibodies drastically reduced the incidence of thymus lymphosarcoma (from ∼ 75% to 30%) in mice exposed to the carcinogens. These data encourage new approaches to the therapy of leukemia by immunological hypophysectomy.

Appendix 1

Endocrine-Induced Regression of Cancers

The natural course can be utterly different in various sorts of malignant disease. Some tumors grow without any apparent restraint whatever. When man harbors a neoplasm of this kind, an increase in the size of the cancer is readily evident from day to day and death ensues in, say, 6 weeks. Conversely, some malignant growths disappear spontaneously. Both of these antipodal effects are rare. Mostly, man with cancer lives 1 year or a little longer after the neoplasm becomes manifest, and it would appear that some inhibition of growth of the tumor takes place to produce this protracted course.

The net increment of mass of a cancer is a function of the interaction of the tumor and its soil. Self-control of cancers results from a highly advantageous competition of host with his tumor. There are multiple factors which restrain cancer—enzymatic, nutritional, immunologic, the genotype, and others. Prominent among them is the endocrine status, both of tumor and host—the subjects of this discourse.

In hormone-responsive cancers, appropriate endocrine modification results in catastrophic effects on cancers of several kinds (Table 1) in man and animals, even in those in the terminal stages of the disease. Of course, there ensues pari passu improvement in the host's condition. The results are often spectacular. The benefit can be evident within a few hours after the intervention. The improvement can persist throughout the re-

The author is William B. Ogden Distinguished Service Professor and Director, Ben May Laboratory for Cancer Research, University of Chicago, Chicago, Illinois 60637. This article is the lecture he delivered in Stockholm, Sweden, 13 December 1966, when he received the Nobel Prize in physiology and medicine which he shared with Francis Peyton Rous. It is published here with the permission of the Nobel Foundation and will also be included in the complete volumes of Nobel lectures in English, published by the Elsevier Publishing Company, Amsterdam and New York.

Table 1   Eight Hormone-Responsive Cancers of Man and Animals

Type of cancer	Species
Carcinoma of breast	Human: female (*17*), male (*18*); rat (*44*)
Carcinoma of prostate	Human (*12*)
Carcinoma of thyroid	Human (*52*)
Lymphosarcoma, leukemia	Mouse (*48*); human (*50*)
Carcinoma of kidney	Hamster (*53*); human (*54*)
Carcinoma of endometrium	Human (*55*)
Carcinoma of seminal vesicle	Human (*56*)
Carcinoma of scent-glands	Hamster (*57*); dog (*58*)

mainder of the life of the organism; in man regressions lasting more than a decade are not uncommon. There can be complete disappearancee of the lesions. But worthwhile benefit ensues only when all or much of the cancer is hormone-responsive and only a small proportion of cancers possess this functional characteristic in pronounced degree.

The therapeutic system of endocrine restraint of cancer came from the efforts of many workers. I was never alone in my studies, in which one or two students always participated as colleagues. It is a privilege to thank the scores of young men and women who sustained our work.

Lacassagne (*1*) was the first to indicate that a correlation probably exists between hormones and the *development* of cancer, since injections of estrone evoked mammary cancer in each of three males of a special strain of mice; carcinoma of the breast had never been observed previously in animals in this category. The proof that hormones can influence the *growth* of cancer was derived from tumors of the prostate of the dog and, later, of man.

The second quarter of our century found the biological sciences much preoccupied with two noble topics: (i) chemistry and physiology of steroids and (ii) biochemistry of organophosphorus compounds. The key to the puzzle of the steroid hormones in cancer was the isolation of crystalline estrone by Doisy *et al.* (*2*) from extracts of urine of pregnant women. In the phosphorus field there were magnificent findings of hexose phosphates, nucleotides, coenzymes and high energy phosphate intermediates. These wonderful discoveries provided the Zeitgeist for our work.

Through the portal of phosphorus metabolism we entered on a series of interconnected observations in steroid endocrinology. A program was not prepared in advance for this basic physiologic study. The work was fascinating and informative so that it provided its own momentum and served as an end in itself. There were blind alleys but eventually the labyrinth of the experimental series was traversed and we were somewhat amazed to find ourselves studying the effects of hormonal status on advanced cancers of people.

Phosphorus Metabolism in Genital Tract

The fluid of spermatocele contains spermatozoa which become motile upon exposure to air. It was observed (*3*) that, remarkably, spermatocele fluid is devoid of acid-soluble phosphorus and free hexoses, whereas human semen contains very large amounts of inorganic phosphorus and a monosaccharide identified as fructose by Mann (*4*). At the time of ejaculation in the human male, the environment of spermatozoa is altered by a sharp rise in its content of fructose and acid soluble phosphorus. We found (*3*) that the seminal vesicle in man is the chief source of these components in semen.

It was somewhat difficult to obtain unmixed secretions from the various accessory sex glands of man, so a simple technique (*5*) was devised to collect the prostatic secretion (Fig. 1) of dogs quantitatively at frequent intervals for years. Often the prostatic fluid of normal adult dogs is secreted for many months with little variation in its quantity or chemical characteristics. This steady state is noteworthy since secretion of the prostate is the end product of a chain of antecedent events involving synthesis of steroids and protein hormones.

Following orchiectomy, the prostate shrinks, the oxidative phase of carbohydrate metabolism declines (*6*), and secretion stops. Testosterone corrects these defects. The cycle of growth and atrophy created by alternately providing and then withholding testosterone was induced repeatedly in the course of the life of the castrate dog. The prostatic cell does not die in the absence of testosterone, it merely shrivels. But the hormone-dependent cancer cell is entirely different. It grows in the presence of supporting hormones but it dies in their absence and for this reason it cannot participate in growth cycles.

A remarkable effect of testosterone is the promotion of growth of its target cells during complete deprival of food. Androstane derivatives conferred on the prostate of puppies a selective nutritional advantage (*7*) during 3 weeks' starvation whereby abundant growth of this gland occurred while there was serious cell breakdown in most of the tissues of the body. It is useless growth since it does not mitigate the ordeal of starvation. It is reminiscent of a nutritional advantage for growth which malignant tumors possess in undernourished hosts. Starvation does not cure cancer.

Hormonal Control of Prostate Cancer

It was good fortune that some of our metabolic experiments had been carried out on dogs since this is the only species of laboratory animal in which tumors of the prostate occur. As in man, it is very common to find spontaneous neoplasms of prostate in aged dogs. Among the signs of great age in this species are cataracts and worn teeth. When testes are present in dogs with these stigmata a prostatic tumor is likely; if, in addition, the dog had an interstital cell tumor of the testis (this was common) a prostatic neoplasm was always found. Most of the canine prostatic tumors are benign growths with much hyperplasia of epithelium and many cysts; carcinoma is usually detected only by histological examination.

At first it was vexatious to encounter a dog with a prostatic tumor during a metabolic study, but before long such dogs were sought. It was soon observed (8) that orchiectomy or the administration of restricted amounts of phenolic estrogens caused a rapid shrinkage of canine prostatic tumors.

The experiments on canine neoplasia proved relevant to human prostate cancer; there had been no earlier reports indicating any relationship of hormones to this malignant growth.

Measurement of phosphatases in blood serum furnished the proof that cancer of the prostate in man is hormone-responsive. The methodology is simple and the results are unequivocal. Kutscher and Wolbergs (9) discovered that acid phosphatase is rich in concentration in the prostate of adult human males. Gutman and Gutman (10) found that many patients with metastatic prostate cancer have significant increases of acid phosphatase in their blood serum. Cancer of the prostate frequently metastasizes to bone where it flourishes and usually evokes proliferation of osteoblasts. In the school of Robert Robison, Kay (11) found that brisk osteoblastic activity gives rise to increased alkaline phosphatase levels in serum.

Human prostate cancer which had metastasized to bone was studied at first. The activities of acid and alkaline phosphatases in the blood were measured concurrently at frequent intervals. The methods are reproducible and not costly in time or materials; both enzymes were measured in duplicate in a small quantity (0.5 ml) of serum. The level of acid phosphatase indicated activity of the disseminated cancer cells in all metastatic loci. The titer of alkaline phosphatase revealed the function of the osteoblasts as influenced by the presence of the prostatic

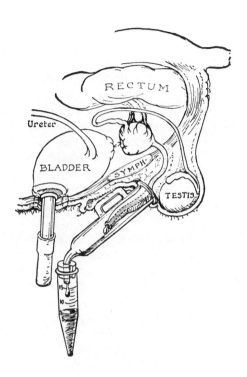

Fig. 1. The prostatic-isolation operation.

cancer cells that were their near neighbors. By periodic measurement of the two enzymes one obtains a view of overall activity of the cancer and the reaction of nonmalignant cells of the host to the presence of that cancer. Thereby the great but opposing influences of, respectively, the administration or deprival of androgenic hormones upon prostate cancer cells were revealed with precision and simplicity. Orchiectomy or the administration of phenolic estrogens resulted in regression of cancer of the human prostate (*12*) whereas, in untreated cases, testosterone enhanced the rate of growth of the neoplasm.

Results consistent with these observations were obtained by studying another enzyme of the prostate, fibrinolysin, in blood of patients with disseminated prostate cancer. In our metabolic studies it had been found that human prostate fluid contained large amounts of many proteolytic enzymes (*13*) and especially one which was highly active against fibrin as a substrate. Prostatic fibrinolysin differs from plasmin and trypsin.

Subsequently Tagnon *et al.* (*14*) observed that the blood of some patients who have metastases of cancer of the prostate becomes incoagulable because of its concentration of prostatic fibrinolysin. The content of this proteolytic enzyme in serum is reduced or eliminated by the administration of estrogenic substances or by gonadectomy; orchiectomy is hazardous when the blood is incoagulable but, fortunately, the pills of diethylstilbestrol are effective therapy. Testosterone causes fibrinolysin to reappear in such patients. The entry of prostatic fibrinolysin into the blood is similar to that of acid phosphatase; each enzyme enters the plasma but only from metastasis and not from the primary neoplasm. The antiandrogenic measures restore the coagulability of the blood.

The control of activity of cancer by excision of endocrine glands is physiologic surgery wherein removal of a normal structure can cause healing of distant disease. Stilbestrol, which had been discovered in 1938 by Dodds *et al.* (*15*), was the first synthetic substance to control cancer; hence the study of the prostate cancers was the start of chemotherapy of malignant disease.

The first series of patients with prostatic cancer treated by orchiectomy (*16*) comprised 21 patients with far advanced metastases; only four of them survived for more than 12 years. Despite regressions of great magnitude, it is obvious that there were many failures of endocrine therapy to control the disease but, on the whole, the life span had been extended by the novel treatments and there had been a decrease of man-pain hours.

Clinical Mammary Cancer

The first indication that advanced cancer can be induced to regress was the beneficial effect of oophorectomy on cancer of the breast in two women. This empirical observation (*17*) of Beatson in 1896 was remarkable since it was made before the concept of hormones had been developed. The beneficial action of removal of ovaries was not understood until steroid hormones had been isolated four decades later.

But why does breast cancer thrive in folks who do not possess ovarian function—in men, old women, and females who have had oophorectomy? Farrow and Adair (*18*) observed that benefits of great magnitude frequently follow orchiectomy in mammary cancer in the human male. Thereby, they established that testis function can sustain mammary cancer.

A half century after the classic invention of Beatson it was found out that adrenal function can maintain and promote growth of human mammary cancer. The adrenal factor supporting growth of cancer was identified (*19*) when it was shown that bilateral adrenalectomy (with glucocorticoids as substitution therapy) can result in profound and prolonged regression of mammary carcinoma in men and women who do not possess gonadal function. In developing the idea of adrenalectomy for treatment of advanced cancer in man we were considerably influenced by the discovery of Woolley·et al. (20) that adrenals can evoke cancer of the breast in the mouse. Regression of great magnitude of human mammary cancer also can be brought about by hypophysectomy (21) as well as by adrenalectomy.

Haddow et al. (22) found that phenolic estrogens can have an ameliorative effect in human mammary cancer. A paradox seemed to be involved since, in some circumstances, estrogenic compounds are activating agents for cancer of the breast. In one room the surgeons were removing sources of estrogenic hormones, while nearby the physicians were prescribing estrogens for mammary cancer; both groups were achieving therapeutic triumphs in some cases. Emerson said, "The ambitious soul sits down before each refractory fact." The vexatious paradox was resolved by experimental studies.

Experimental Mammary Cancer

Many of the early investigations in this area were carried out in mice and admirable discoveries had been made; chiefly, these concerned the etiology of mammary cancer. But there was a serious disadvantage in use of the mouse—mammary cancers in this species are seldom hormone-responsive. True, in some strains breast cancer diminished somewhat during lactation (23) and increased in size during pregnancy. But Mühlbock (24) found that in most strains of mice mammary cancers are hormone-independent when the tumors have reached palpable size. Yet the thing about cancers is to cure them.

Studies of the rat altered the course of research on breast cancer because this species has a remarkable propensity to develop mammary carcinoma after exposure to aromatics or, to a lesser extent, irradiation. Further, many of the cancers of rat evoked by these methods are completely hormone-dependent and so can be extinguished by endocrine methods.

Compared with mouse and other rodents, rat is extremely vulnerable (25) to polynuclear aromatic hydrocarbons. In the rat, small amounts of carcinogenic aromatics exert the following effects: (i) profound depression of incorporation (25) of thymidine in DNA; (ii) augmented production of messenger RNA (26); (iii) induction of synthesis of a soluble enzyme, menadione reductase (27) and of microsome-bound enzymes and other proteins (28); (iv) cause cancer or death of the recipient (29). Maisin and Coolen (30) repeatedly painted mice with 3-methylcholanthrene and observed that, in addition to cancer of the skin, mammary cancer developed in a small but significant percentage of the animals after 7 months. Shay (31) fed rats a small dose of 3-methylcholanthrene each day for many months and observed a high incidence of mammary cancer; the tumors were first detected after 4 months. We found that, under conditions which are highly restricted but easily satisfied, a single massive but tolerable dose of any of a large number (*32*) of polynuclear aromatic hydrocarbons or aromatic amines rapidly and selectively induced breast cancers which were palpable within 1 month. It is a method of extreme simplicity. Two carcinogenic aromatics, 7,8,12-trimethyl- and 7,12-dimethylbenz-(a)anthracene are ten times more efficient than all others.

Whereas a single feeding of a solution of 7,12-dimethylbenz-(a)anthracene always induces breast tumors (*33*), intravenous injection of a concentrated lipid emulsion (*34*) of the aromatic is equally efficacious and has an additional advantage—it introduces the compounds suddenly into the blood as a pulse-dose. When three pulse-doses of 7,12-dimethylbenz(a)anthracene were given to Sprague-Dawley female rats, at age 50, 53, and 56 days, mammary tumors were evoked in all animals and large numbers of breast cancers (*35*) were palpable within 4 weeks. The superficial location of rat's mammary glands readily permits detection of the cancers by palpation and the end point is sharp because the cancers are firm in consistency and discrete. A tumor weighing 8 to 10 mg can be detected with ease. The earliest mammary cancer was found by histological search on day 11 and by palpation on day 20 after the pulse-dose. This is somewhat comparable to a famous experiment of Rous (*36*) who injected a cell-free filtrate of chicken sarcoma I into other fowls and observed the first palpable tumor 10 to 21 days thereafter. In contradistinction to the Rous virus, aromatic hydrocarbons elicit benign tumors of the breast in addition to the cancers.

The mammary cancers of the rat seldom metastasize but kill the host by attaining great size and invading adjacent tissues. Metastases can be produced readily; in the experiment of Dao (*37*) injection of mammary cancer cells in portal vein caused multiple cancers in the liver. The respiration values (*38*) of the mammary cancers are similar to those of normal lactating mammary gland. The high rate of glycolysis, which Warburg (*39*) found to be distinctive of the metabolism of cancer, prevailed in the induced carcinomas.

Rats are also rather susceptible to the development of mammary cancer after exposure to a big dose of ionizing radiation (*40*). Both 7,12-dimethylbenz(a)anthracene (*41*) and radiation (*42*) possess the ability to inflict selective lesions of identical sort in rat's testis. With these agents the prime targets are those germinal cells which multiply by mitosis and hence synthesize DNA; in contrast, those cells of testis which proliferate by meiosis and do not synthesize DNA are spared from injury.

Hormone-Deprival in Control of Cancer

Mammary cancers induced in the male rat by aromatics were not influenced by orchiectomy and hypophysectomy (*43*); by definition, these neoplasms are hormone-independent. In contrast to male rat, most mammary cancers of men wither impressively after deprival of supporting hormones.

The hormone-responsiveness of established mammary cancers induced in female rat by aromatics (*44*) or ionizing radiation (*45*) is identical; it was a newly recognized property of experimental breast cancers. Prior to this finding, clinical study of patients with mammary cancer was the only avenue available for investigation of hormonal-restraint of neoplasms of the breast.

In female rat, growth of the mammary cancers was accelerated in pregnancy and by progestational compounds (*46*). We have not found any dosage of estradiol-17β which markedly enhanced the growth of these tumors.

In female rat, many but far from all of the induced mammary cancers vanished after removal of ovaries or the pituitary. In our experiments hypophysectomy was the most efficient of all methods to cure rat's mammary cancer. Malignant cells which succumb to hormone-deprival, by definition, are hormone-dependent. The quality of hormone-dependence resides in the tumor cells whereas their growth is determined by the host's endocrine status. Both man and the animals can have some of their cancer cells which are hormone-dependent while other neoplastic cells in the same organism are not endocrine-responsive.

The cure of a cancer after hormone-deprival results from death of the cancer cells, whereas their normal analogues in the same animal shrivel but survive. It is a basic proposition in endocrine-restraint of malignant disease that cancer cells can differ in a crucial way from ancestral normal cells in response to modification of the hormonal *milieu intérieur* of the body.

Hormone-Interference in Cancer Control

It was unexpected to find that mammary cancers can be extinguished by providing excessive amounts of ovarian steroids; this effect is cancer control by hormone-interference.

We induced mammary carcinoma in rats which were then treated for a limited time with large amounts of estradiol plus progesterone (*46*). This combination of hormones excited such exuberant growth of normal mammary cells that the breasts resembled those of rats late in pregnancy. Nevertheless, many of the mammary cancers were completely eliminated, and 52 percent of the rats were free from cancer (*32*) 6 months after steroids had been discontinued. These rats had been cured of cancer because the tumors did not reappear during subsequent pregnancy. The heavy hormonal burden of pregnancy upon mammary cancer had not reactivated dormant cancer cells if any had been present.

In patients, the combination of huge amounts of progesterone and of estradiol, injected intramuscularly, induced measurable and worthwhile improvement (*47*) in patients with far advanced disseminated mammary cancer, both in women and men. Moreover, benefit was obtained in patients in whom other forms of endocrine therapy such as adrenalectomy and oophorectomy had previously promoted tumor regression followed by recrudescence.

In another type of hormone-interference, cancer cells are exterminated in parallel with normal cells of similar kind. Glucocorticoids will cause a remission of some chronic lymphogenous tumors and leukemia. Heilman and Kendall administered large amounts of cortisone to mice bearing a transplanted lymphosarcoma: "Although dramatic and apparently complete cures are produced, they are only temporary in a majority of animals" (*48*). In contrast to the beneficial effects of cortisone, adrenalectomy enhances growth of lymphomas in mouse (*49*). Pearson *et al.* (*50*) found that corticotropin or cortisone caused dramatic if temporary regression in certain cases of human leukemia and Hodgkin's disease.

Dougherty and White (*51*) found that administration of pituitary corticotropin (ACTH) to the mouse causes a regression of lymph nodes and thymus. Regression of lymphomas brought about by glucocorticoids does not differ in principle from the effect of corticosteroids on the lymphocytes of normal animals and man.

Conclusions

Cancer is not necessarily autonomous and intrinsically self-perpetuating. Its growth can be sustained and propagated by hormonal function in the host which is not unusual in kind or exaggerated in rate but which is operating at normal or even subnormal levels.

Hormones, or synthetic substances inducing physiologic effects similar thereto, are of crucial significance for survival of several kinds of hormone-responsive cancers in man and animals. Opposite sorts of change of the hormonal status can induce regression and, in some instances, cure such cancers. These modifications are deprivation of essential hormones and hormone interference by giving large amounts of critical compounds.

The control of cancer by endocrine methods can be described in three propositions: (i) Some types of cancer cells differ in a cardinal way from the cells from which they arose in their response to change in their hormonal environment. (ii) Certain cancers are hormone-dependent and these cells die when supporting hormones are eliminated. (iii) Certain cancers succumb when large amounts of hormones are administered.

References

1. A. Lacassagne, *Compt. Rend.* 195, 630 (1932).
2. E. A. Doisy, C. D. Veler, S. Thayer, *Amer. J. Physiol.* 90, 329 (1929).
3. C. B. Huggins and A. A. Johnson, *ibid.* 103, 574 (1933).
4. T. Mann, *Biochemistry of Semen and of the Male Reproductive Tract* (Methuen, London, 1964).
5. C. Huggins, M. H. Masina, L. Eichelberger, J. D. Wharton, *J. Exp. Med.* 70, 543 (1939).
6. E. S. G. Barron and C. Huggins, *J. Urol.* 51, 630 (1944).
7. R. Pazos, Jr., and C. Huggins, *Endocrinology* 36, 416 (1945).
8. C. Huggins and P. J. Clark, *J. Exp. Med.* 72, 747 (1940).
9. W. Kutscher and H. Wolbergs, *Z. Physiol. Chem.* 236, 237 (1940).
10. A. B. Gutman and E. B. Gutman, *J. Clin. Invest.* 17, 473 (1938).
11. H. D. Kay, *Brit. J. Exp. Pathol* 10, 253 (1929).
12. C. Huggins and C. V. Hodges, *Cancer Res.* 1, 293 (1941).
13. C. Huggins and W. Neal, *J. Exp. Med.* 76, 527 (1942).
14. H. J. Tagnon, W. F. Whitmore, Jr., N. R. Shulman, *Cancer* 5, 9 (1952).
15. E. C. Dodds, L. Golberg, W. Lawson, R. Robinson, *Proc. Roy. Soc. London, Ser. B* 127, 140 (1939).
16. C. Huggins, R. E. Stevens, Jr., C. V. Hodges, *Arch. Surg.* 43, 209 (1941).
17. G. T. Beatson, *Lancet* 1896–II, 104, 162 (1896).
18. J. H. Farrow and F. E. Adair, *Science* 95, 654 (1942).
19. C. Huggins and D. M. Bergenstal, *Cancer Res.* 12, 134 (1952).
20. G. W. Woolley, E. Fekete, C. C. Little, *Proc. Nat. Acad. Sci. U.S.* 25, 277 (1939).
21. R. Luft, H. Olivecrona, B. Sjögren, *Nord Med.* 47, 351 (1952).
22. A. Haddow, J. M. Watkinson, E. Paterson, *Brit. Med. J.* 2, 393 (1944).
23. A. Haddow, *J. Pathol. Bacteriol.* 47, 553 (1938); F. Bielschowsky, *Brit. Med. Bull.* 4, 382 (1947); L. Foulds, *Brit. J. Cancer* 3, 345 (1949).
24. O. Mühlbock, in *Endocrine Aspects of Breast Cancer*, A. R. Currie, Ed. (Livingstone, Edinburgh, 1958), p. 291.
25. C. B. Huggins, E. Ford, E. V. Jensen, *Science* 147, 1153 (1965).
26. L. A. Loeb and H. V. Gelboin, *Proc. Nat. Acad. Sci. U.S.* 52, 1219 (1964).

27. H. G. Williams-Ashman and C. Huggins, *Med. Exp.* 4, 223 (1961).
28. J. C. Arcos, A. H. Conney, N. P. Buu-Hoi, *J. Biol. Chem.* 236, 1291 (1961).
29. C. Huggins and R. Fukunishi, *J. Exp. Med.* 119, 923 (1964).
30. J. Maisin and M.-L. Coolen, *Compt. Rend. Soc. Biol.* 123, 159 (1936).
31. H. Shay, *et al., J. Nat. Cancer Inst.* 10, 255 (1949).
32. C. Huggins and N. C. Yang, *Science* 137, 257 (1962).
33. C. Huggins, L. C. Grand, F. P. Brillantes, *Nature* 189, 204 (1961).
34. R. P. Geyer, J. E. Bryant, V. R. Bleisch, E. M. Peirce, F. J. Stare, *Cancer Res.* 13, 503 (1953); C. Huggins, S. Morii, L. C. Grand, *Ann. Surg.* 154 (Suppl.) 315 (1961).
35. C. Huggins, L. Grand, R. Fukunishi, *Proc. Nat. Acad. Sci. U.S.* 51, 737 (1964).
36. P. Rous, *J. Exp. Med.* 13, 397 (1911).
37. T. L. Dao, *Progr. Exp. Tumor Res.* 5, 157 (1964).
38. E. D. Rees and C. Huggins, *Cancer Res.* 20, 963 (1960).
39. O. Warburg, *Metabolism of Tumours* (Constable, London, 1930).
40. J. G. Hamilton, P. W. Durbin, M. Parrott, *J. Clin. Endocrinol.* 14, 1161 (1954); C. J. Shellabarger, E. P. Cronkite, V. P. Bond, S. W. Lippincott, *Radiation Res.* 6, 501 (1957).
41. E. Ford and C. Huggins, *J. Exp. Med.* 118, 27 (1963).
42. C. Regaud and J. Blanc, *Compt. Rend. Soc. Biol.* 58, 163 (1906).
43. C. Huggins and L. C. Grand, *Cancer Res.* 26, 2255 (1966).
44. C. Huggins, G. Briziarelli, H. Sutton, Jr., *J. Exp. Med.* 109, 25 (1959).
45. C. Huggins and R. Fukunishi, *Radiation Res.* 20, 493 (1963).
46. C. Huggins, R. C. Moon, S. Morii, *Proc. Nat. Acad. Sci. U.S.* 48, 379 (1962).
47. R. L. Landau, E. N. Ehrlich, C. Huggins, *J. Amer. Med. Ass.* 182, 632 (1962); L. G. Crowley and I. Macdonald, *Cancer* 18, 436 (1965); B. J. Kennedy, *ibid.,* p. 1551.
48. F. R. Heilman and E. C. Kendall, *Endocrinology* 34, 416 (1944).
49. J. B. Murphy and E. Sturm, *Science* 98, 568 (1943).
50. O. H. Pearson, L. P. Eliel, R. W. Rawson, K. Dobriner, C. P. Rhoads, *Cancer* 2, 943 (1949).
51. T. F. Dougherty and A. White, *Proc. Soc. Exp. Biol. Med.* 55, 132 (1943).
52. H. W. Balme, *Lancet* 1954 I, 812 (1954); G. Crile, Jr., *J. Amer. Med. Ass.* 195, 721 (1966).
53. H. Kirkman, *Nat. Cancer Inst. Monogr.* 1, 1 (1959).
54. H. J. G. Bloom, C. E. Dukes, B. C. V. Mitchley, *Brit J. Cancer* 17, 611 (1963).
55. R. M. Kelley and W. H. Baker, *New Engl. J. Med.* 264, 216 (1961).
56. O. S. Rodriguez Kees, *J. Urol.* 91, 665 (1964).
57. H. Kirkman and F. T. Algard, *Cancer Res.* 24, 1569 (1964).
58. S. W. Nielsen and J. Aftsomis, *J. Amer. Vet. Med. Ass.* 144, 127 (1964).
59. This investigation was aided by grants from the Jane Coffin Childs Memorial Fund for Medical Research and the American Cancer Society. The Upjohn Company, Kalamazoo, Michigan, through P. Schurr, provided the lipid emulsions of hydrocarbons.

Appendix 2

Composition and Preparation of Experimental Intravenous Fat Emulsions

by Paul E. Schurr

Summary

Components and procedures used to prepare intravenous fat emulsions for animal experiments are described. These are exemplified by details for making the emulsions containing 7,12-dimethylbenz(a)anthracene used to induce mammary cancer and leukemia.

Introduction

An extensive review of the literature concerning composition, preparation, metabolism, and clinical utilization of intravenous fat emulsions has been published by Geyer (2). Of the various preparations proposed for clinical use, a 15% cottonseed oil emulsion stabilized with purified soybean lecithin and Pluronic-F68 (Lipomul®-I.V., The Upjohn Company) (12) was studied most extensively in animals and man. It was found to be well tolerated by animals and humans during short-term administrations, but the possibility of the development of a "long-term reaction" (14) in humans receiving multiple infusions necessitated restrictions in its use (13, 14). Although Lipomul®-I.V. is no longer available for use in humans, The Upjohn Company has prepared experimental emulsions for animal use in studies of lipid metabolism and as vehicles for parenteral administration of fat soluble agents. Most notable examples are the emulsions containing the carcinogen 7,12-dimethylbenz(a)anthracene (DMBA), made a popular tool for cancer research by Huggins (6, 7). The present communication details the methods used in preparing DMBA emulsions at The Upjohn Company so that they may be duplicated by other laboratories. With appropriate changes in composition these procedures also apply to other experimental emulsions.

Reprinted by permission from *Cancer Research* 29 (January 1969): 258–60.

The author is in Cardiovascular Diseases Research, the Upjohn Company, Kalamazoo.

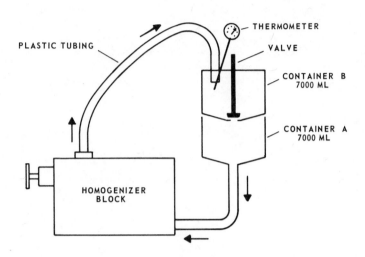

Chart 1. Diagram of high-pressure homogenizing system used in preparing i.v. fat emulsions.

Process. The DMBA was dissolved in the lecithin and oil on a steam bath. The Pluronic F-68 was dissolved in about 200 ml of water at room temperature and then added to the rest of the water preheated to 75°C. The water phase was poured into container A and the homogenizer adjusted to 3000 psi. By appropriate direction of the discharge, a vortex was created and the oil phase at 70 ± 2°C was poured slowly into its center. After the oil was added, container B was placed in the system and cycling of the homogenate continued for a total of 2 min. Then the valve in container B was closed until about 4 liters of homogenate had collected; this was then released to container A by opening the valve. The homogenate was cycled in this manner a total of 3 times. During the process the homogenate was kept from exceeding 72°C by cooling the homogenizer block with crushed ice or cold water. After the 3rd cycle, the emulsion was discharged into a side-container until air entered the pump. The last 200–300 ml contained in the pump were discarded.

Packaging. We preferred filling small vials from a 3 liter separatory funnel, keeping at least 1 liter in it until the last, to prevent contamination by the foam and accompanying large fat particles. Containers were filled to about 80% of capacity, to allow for increased vapor pressure during sterilization.

Sterilization and Cooling. The emulsions were autoclaved at 121°C for 15 min. After sterilization the autoclave was adjusted to reach atmospheric pressure rapidly (within 10 min). As soon as possible, with adequate safety precautions, the bottles were agitated while in the autoclave to prevent refluxing on the upper surfaces of the bottles. Within 5 minutes the bottles were removed and cooled as rapidly as possible to 5°C with shaking. Small bottles (20–100 ml) were cooled within 15 min by turning a fan on them for about 5 min and then spraying with hot water, followed by progressively cooler water, and finally iced water. Larger bottles require more time under the fan before spraying. The emulsions were stored in the dark at 5°C.

Evaluation of Emulsion

The physical qualities of emulsions were judged by microscopic examination of undiluted samples. The bottle of emulsion was inverted, not shaken, at least 3 times, and 1 drop of emulsion was placed in each chamber of a Spencer Bright Line Improved Neubauer hemocytometer. Precautions were taken to prevent contact of the pipet with the hemocytometer, since any disturbance of the cover slip caused air bubbles and/or coalescence of emulsion particles. Fat particles with diameters $>7-14$ μ were counted within the lined (9 sq mm) area of each chamber, using low magnification ($\times$ 100) and a calibrated eye-piece scale. Using this technic, satisfactory emulsions had average counts per chamber of 40 particles >7 μ in diameter and thirteen >14 μ. These counts vary by about 50%; however, poor emulsions were easily indicated by more than twofold increases in counts. We have also evaluated the emulsions by oil immersion light microscopy and electronic (Coulter) counting (16). By these procedures it was estimated that about 97% of the oil was in emulsion particles ≤ 1 μ in diameter (mean <0.01 μ). Particles ≥ 5 μ were rarely noted. These methods provide reliable estimates of the size distributions of smaller emulsion particles but not of larger sizes. We rely almost exclusively upon evaluating by hemocytometer to indicate emulsion quality. Generally, ability to evaluate by this method indicates that the bulk of emulsion particles were ≤ 1 μ, since emulsions containing large percentages of particles > 1 μ do not transmit light in the hemocytometer.

Discussion

The method and materials used to produce emulsions with small particle sizes and remarkable stability have been described. When less satisfactory emulsions are obtained, the difficulty can usually be traced to homogenizing with worn valves or air trapped in the system, cycling completed emulsion under reduced pressure, or failure to minimize evaporation from the surface of the emulsion after sterilization. Although 3- to 6-kg lots were generally prepared by this procedure, the method may be

References

Abercrombie, M. 1961. Behaviour of normal and malignant connective tissue cells *in vitro*. *Canadian Cancer Conference* 4:101–17. New York: Academic Press.

Ames, B. N., Durston, W. E., Yamasaki, E., and Lee, F. D. 1973. Carcinogens are mutagens: A simple test system combining liver homogenates for activation and bacteria for detection. *Proc. Natl. Acad. Sci. USA* 70:2281–85.

Ames, B. N., Lee, F. D., and Durston, W. E. 1973. An improved bacterial test system and classification of mutagens and carcinogens. *Proc. Natl. Acad. Sci. USA* 70:782–86.

Andervont, H. B. 1940. The influence of foster nursing upon the incidence of spontaneous mammary cancer in resistant and susceptible mice. *J. Natl. Cancer Inst.* 1:147–53.

Arcos, J. C., Conney, A. H., and Buu-Hoi, N. P. 1961. Induction of microsomal enzyme synthesis by polycyclic aromatic hydrocarbons of different molecular sizes. *J. Biol. Chem.* 236: 1291–96.

Aub, J. C., Sanford, B. H., and Wang, L.-H. 1965. Reactions of normal and leukemic cell surfaces to a wheat germ agglutinin. *Proc. Natl. Acad. Sci. USA* 54: 400–402.

Aub, J. C., Tieslau, C., and Lankester, A. 1963. Reactions of normal and tumor cell surfaces to enzymes. I. Wheat-germ lipase and associated mucopolysaccharides. *Proc. Natl. Acad. Sci. USA* 50:613–19.

Bachmann, W. E., and Chemerda, J. M. 1938. The synthesis of 9,10-dimethyl-1,2-benzanthracene, 9,10-diethyl-1,2-benzanthracene and 5,9,10-trimethyl-1,2-benzanthracene. *J. Am. Chem. Soc.* 60:1023–26.

Bachmann, W. E., Cook, J. W., Dansi, A., DeWorms, C. G. M., Haslewood, G. A. D., Hewett, C. L., and Robinson, A. M. 1937. The production of cancer by pure hydrocarbons. IV. *Proc. Roy. Soc. B.* 123:343–68.

Boyland, E., and Sims, P. 1965. Metabolism of polycyclic compounds. The metabolism of 7,12-dimethylbenz[a]anthracene by rat-liver homogenates. *Biochem. J.* 95:780–87.

Boyland, E., Sims, P., and Huggins, C. B. 1965. Induction of adrenal damage and cancer with metabolites of 7,12-dimethylbenz[a]anthracene. *Nature* 207:816–17.

Brand, K. G., Buoen, L. C., and Brand, I. 1969. Premalignant cells in tumorigenesis induced by plastic films. *Nature* 213: 810.

Brodie, B. B., Axelrod, J., Cooper, J. R., Gaudette, L., LaDu, B. N., Mitoma, C., and Udenfriend, S. 1955. Detoxication of drugs and other foreign compounds by liver microsomes. *Science* 121:603–4.

Broome, J. D. 1963. Evidence that the L-asparaginase of guinea pig serum is responsible for its antilymphoma effects. *J. Exptl Med.* 118:99–120.

Bryan, W. R., and Shimkin, M. B. 1943. Quantitative analysis of dose response data obtained with three carcinogenic hydrocarbons in strain C3H male mice. *J. Natl. Cancer Inst.* 3: 503–31.

Burger, M. M. 1969. A difference in the architecture of the surface membrane of normal and virally transformed cells. *Proc. Natl. Acad. Sci. USA* 62:994–1001.

Burger, M. M., and Goldberg, A. R. 1967. Identification of a tumor-specific determinant on neoplastic cell surfaces. *Proc. Natl. Acad. Sci. USA* 57:359–66.

Burn, J. H., Finney, D. J., and Goodwin, L. G. 1950. *Biological Standardization*, p. 114. 2d ed. London: Oxford University Press.

Burrows, H., Hieger, I., and Kennaway, E. L. 1932. The experimental production of tumours of connective tissue. *Am. J. Cancer* 16:57–67.

Bush, I. E. 1953. Species differences in adrenocortical secretion. *J. Endocrinol.* 9:95–100.

Butenandt, A., and Kudszus, H. 1935. Über Androstendion, einen hochwirksamen mannlichen Prägungsstoff. *Z. physiol. Chem.* 237:75–88.

Cade, S. 1955. Adrenalectomy for breast cancer. *Brit. Med. J.* 1:1–4.

Cantarow, A., Stasney, J., and Paschkis, K. E. 1948. The influence of sex hormones on mammary tumors induced by 2-acetylaminofluorene. *Cancer Res.* 8:412–17.

Capizzi, R. L., Peterson, R., Cooney, D. A., Creasey, W. A., and Handschumacher, R. E. 1969. L-asparaginase therapy of acute leukemia: biochemical and clinical observations. *Proc. Am. Assoc. Cancer Res.* 10:12.

Cardiff, R. D., Blair, P. B., and DeOme, K. B. 1968. *In vitro* cultivation of the mouse mammary tumor virus: replication of MTV in tissue culture. *Virology* 36:313–17.

Cartland, G. F., and Nelson, J. W. 1937. The preparation and purification of extracts containing the gonad-stimulating hormone of pregnant mare serum. *J. Biol. Chem.* 119:59–67.

Cartland, G. F., and Nelson, J. W. 1938. The bioassay of mare serum hormone. A comparison of ovarian and uterine weight methods. *Am. J. Physiol.* 122:201–6.

Clemens, J. A., Welsch, C. W., and Meites, J. 1968. Effects of hypothalamic lesions on incidence and growth of mammary tumors in carcinogen-treated rats. *Proc. Soc. Exptl. Biol. Med.* 127:969–72.

Clermont, Y., Leblond, C. P., and Messier, B. 1959. Durée du cycle de l'epithélium séminal du rat. *Arch. Anat. Micr.* 48: 37–55.

Conney, A. H., and Burns, J. J. 1959. Stimulatory effect of foreign compounds on ascorbic acid biosynthesis and on drug-metabolizing enzymes. *Nature* (London) 184:363–64.

Conney, A. H., and Klutch, A. 1963. Increased activity of androgen hydroxylases in liver of rats pretreated with phenobarbital and other drugs. *J. Biol. Chem.* 238:1611–17.

Conney, A. H., Miller, E. C., and Miller, J. A. 1956. The metabolism of methylated aminoazo dyes. V. Evidence for induction of enzyme synthesis in the rat by 3-methylcholanthrene. *Cancer Res.* 16:450–59.

Conney, A. H., Miller, E. C., and Miller, J. A. 1957. Substrate-induced synthesis and other properties of benzpyrene hydroxylase in rat liver. *J. Biol. Chem.* 228:753–56.

Cook, J. W. 1932. The production of cancer by pure hydrocarbons—Part II. *Proc. Royal Soc. London, B* 111:485–96.

Cook, J. W. 1958. Ernest Laurance Kennaway. *Biographical Memoirs of Fellows of the Royal Society* 4:139–54.

Cook, J. W., Hewett, C. L., and Hieger, I. 1933. The isolation of a cancer-producing hydrocarbon from coal tar. *J. Chem. Soc.* 395–405.

Cook, J. W., Hieger, I., Kennaway, E. L., and Mayneord, W. V. 1932. The production of cancer by pure hydrocarbons—Part I. *Proc. Royal Soc. London, B* 111:455–84.

Cori, C. F. 1927. The influence of ovariectomy on the spontaneous occurrence of mammary carcinomas in mice. *J. Exptl. Med.* 45:983–91.

Dunning, W. F., and Curtis, M. R. 1960. Relative carcinogenicity of monomethyl derivatives of benz[*a*]anthracene in Fischer line 344 rats. *J. Natl. Cancer Inst.* 25:387–91.

Dunning, W. F., Curtis, M. R., and Segaloff, A. 1947. Strain differences in response to diethylstilbestrol and the induction of mammary gland and bladder cancer in the rat. *Cancer Res.* 7:511–21.

Earle, W. R. and Nettleship, A. 1943. Production of malignancy *in vitro*. V. Results of injections of cultures into mice. *J. Natl. Cancer Inst.* 4:213–227.

Eckhart, W. 1969. Cell transformation by polyoma virus and SV40. *Nature* 224: 1069–71.

Edwards, J. L., and Klein, R. E. 1961. Cell renewal in adult mouse tissues. *Am. J. Pathol.* 38:437–53.

Ellermann, V., and Bang, O. 1908. Experimentelle Leukämie bei Hühnern. *Centr. Bakt.* 66:595–609.

Ellermann, V., and Bang, O. 1909. Experimentelle Leukämie bei Hühnern. II. *Z. Hygiene* 63:231–72.

Engelbreth-Holm, J. 1941. Acceleration of the development of mammary carcinomas in mice by methylcholanthrene. *Cancer Res.* 1:109–12.

Ernster, L., Ljunggren, M., and Danielson, L. 1960. Purification and some properties of a highly dicumarol-sensitive liver diaphorase. *Biochem. Biophys. Res. Comm.* 2:88–92.

Estabrook, R. W., Cooper, D. Y., and Rosenthal, O. 1963. The light-reversible carbon monoxide inhibition of the steroid C21-hydroxylase system of the adrenal cortex. *Biochem. Z.* 338:741–55.

Ferguson, D. J., and Visscher, M. B. 1953. The effect of hypophysectomy on the development of adrenal tumors in C3H mice. *Cancer Res.* 13:405–7.

Fernö, O., Fex, H., Högberg, B., Linderrot, T., Veige, S., and Diczfalusy, E. 1958. III. High molecular weight enzyme inhibitors. Polyestradiol phosphate (P.E.P.) a long-acting estrogen. *Acta Chem. Scand.* 12:1675–89.

Fiebig, H.-H., and Schmähl, D. 1978. Effect of ovariectomy, ergocornin and tamoxifen alone or in combination on chemically induced mammary cancer of the rat. In: *Current Chemotherapy*, edited by W. Siegenthaler and R. Lüthy, pp. 1283–85. Washington: American Society for Microbiology.

Fieser, L. F., and Hershberg, E. B. 1937. Aceanthrene derivatives related to cholanthrene. *J. Am. Chem. Soc.* 59:394–98.

Fieser, L. F., and Newman, M. S. 1936. The synthesis of 1,2-

benzanthracene derivatives related to cholanthrene. *J. Am. Chem. Soc.* 58:2376–82.

Fieser, L. F., and Seligman, A. M. 1935*a*. The synthesis of methylcholanthrene. *J. Am. Chem. Soc.* 57:942–46.

Fieser, L. F., and Seligman, A. M. 1935*b*. Cholanthrene and related hydrocarbons. *J. Am. Chem. Soc.* 57:2174–76.

Fischer, B. 1906. Die experimentelle Erzeugung atypischer Epithelwucherungen und die Entstehung bosartiger Geschwülste. *Muench. med. Wochschr.* 53:2041–47.

Ford, E., and Huggins, C. B. 1963. Selective destruction in testis induced by 7,12-dimethylbenz[*a*]anthracene. *J. Exptl. Med.* 118:27–40.

Foster, R. 1969. *Organic Charge-Transfer Complexes.* New York: Academic Press.

Friderichsen, C. 1955. Waterhouse-Friderichsen syndrome (W.-F.S.). *Acta Endocrinol.* 18:482–92.

Friend, C. 1957. Cell-free transmission in adult Swiss mice of a disease having the characteristics of a leukemia. *J. Exptl. Med.* 105:307–18.

Friend, C., Scher, W., Holland, J. G., and Sato, T. 1971. Hemoglobin synthesis in murine virus-induced leukemic cells *in vitro:* Stimulation of erythroid differentiation by dimethyl sulfoxide. *Proc. Natl. Acad. Sci. USA* 68:378–82.

Fukuhara, S., Shirakawa, S., and Uchino, H. 1976. Specific marker chromosome 14 in malignant lymphomas. *Nature* 259:210–11.

Furth, J., and Burnett, Jr., W. T. 1951. Hormone-secreting transplantable neoplasms of the pituitary induced by I[131]. *Proc. Soc. Exptl. Biol. Med.* 78:222–24.

Gardner, W. U. 1948. Hormonal imbalances in tumorigenesis *Cancer Res.* 8:397–411.

Gardner, W. U., Dougherty, T. F., and Williams, W. L. 1944. Lymphoid tumors in mice receiving steroid hormones. *Cancer Res.* 4:73–87.

Gardner, W. U., and White, A. 1941. Mammary growth in hypophysectomized male mice receiving estrogen and prolactin. *Proc. Soc. Exptl. Biol. Med.* 48:590–92.

Gelboin, H. V., and Blackburn, N. R. 1964. The stimulatory effect of 3-methylcholanthrene on benzpyrene hydroxylase activity in several rat tissues: Inhibition by actinomycin D and puromycin. *Cancer Res.* 24:356–60.

Geyer, R. P., Bleisch, V. R., Bryant, J. E., Robbins, A. N., Saslaw, I. M., and Stare, F. J. 1951. Tumor production in rats injected intravenously with oil emulsions containing 9,10-dimethyl-1,2-benzanthracene. *Cancer Res.* 11:474–78.

Geyer, R. P., Bryant, J. E., Bleisch, V. R., Peirce, E. M., and Stare, F. J. 1953. Effect of dose and hormones on tumor production in rats given emulsified 9,10-dimethyl-1,2-benzanthracene intravenously. *Cancer Res.* 13:503–6.

Goldman, R. D., Kaplan, N. O., and Hall, T. C. 1964. Lactic dehydrogenase in human neoplastic tissues. *Cancer Res* 24:389–99.

Gorbman, A. 1950. Functional and structural changes consequent to high dosages of radioactive iodine. *J. Clin. Endocrinol.* 10:1177–91.

Gordon, A. S. 1954. Endocrine influences upon the formed elements of the blood and blood-forming organs. *Recent Progr Hormone Res.* 10:339–94.

Green, H., Todaro, G. J., and Goldberg, B. 1966. Collagen synthesis in fibroblasts transformed by oncogenic viruses. *Nature* 209:916–17.

Greenstein, J. P. 1947. *Biochemistry of Cancer.* New York Academic Press.

Gross, L. 1950. Susceptibility of newborn mice of an otherwise "resistant" strain to inoculation with leukemia. *Proc. Soc Exptl. Biol. Med.* 73:246–48.

Gross, L. 1951. "Spontaneous" leukemia developing in C3H mice following inoculation in infancy with Ak-leukemic extracts, or Ak-embryos. *Proc. Soc. Exptl. Biol. Med.* 76:27–32.

Gross, L. 1957. Development and serial cell-free passage of a highly potent strain of mouse leukemia virus. *Proc. Soc Exptl. Biol. Med.* 94:767–71.

Gross, L. 1961a. Induction of leukemia in rats with mouse leukemia (Passage A) virus. *Proc. Soc. Exptl. Biol. Med* 106:890–93.

Gross, L. 1961b. *Oncogenic Viruses,* pp. 281. New York: Pergamon Press.

Gruenstein, M., Meranze, D. R., Thatcher, D., and Shimkin M. B. 1966. Carcinogenic effects of intragastric 3-methylcholanthrene and 7,12-dimethylbenz[a]anthracene in Wistar and Sprague-Dawley rats. *J. Natl. Cancer Inst.* 36:483–502.

Guillemin, R., Clayton, G. W., Lipscomb, H. S., and Smith J. D. 1959. Fluorometric measurement of rat plasma and adrenal corticosterone concentration; a note on technical details. *J. Lab. Clin. Med.* 53:830–32.

Gullino, P. M., Pettigrew, H. M., and Grantham, F. H. 1975

N-Nitrosomethylurea as mammary gland carcinogen in rats. *J. Natl. Cancer Inst.* 54:401–9.

Haagensen, C. D., and Randall, H. T. 1942. Production of mammary carcinoma in mice by estrogens. *Arch. Pathol.* 33:411–22.

Haddow, A., Harris, R. J. C., Kon, G. A. R., and Roe, E. M. F. 1948. The growth-inhibitory and carcinogenic properties of 4-aminostilbene and derivatives. *Phil. Trans. Royal Soc. London.* A 241:147–95.

Haddow, A., Watkinson, J. M., Paterson, E., and Koller, P. C. 1944. Influence of synthetic oestrogens upon advanced malignant disease. *Brit. Med. J.* 2:393–98.

Hamilton, J. G., Durbin, P. W., and Parrott, M. 1954. The accumulation and destructive action of Astatine[211] (*eka*-iodine) in the thyroid glands of rats and monkeys. *J. Clin. Endocrinol. Metab.* 14:1161–78.

Haran-Ghera, N., Kotler, M., and Meshorer, A. 1967. Studies on leukemia development in the SJL/J strain of mice. *J. Natl. Cancer Inst.* 39:653–61.

Hartmann, H. A., Miller, E. C., Miller, J. A., and Morris, F. K. 1959. The leukemogenic action of 2-acetylaminophenanthrene in the rat. *Cancer Res.* 19:210–216.

Haugen, D. A., Coon, M. J., and Nebert, D. W. 1976. Induction of multiple forms of mouse liver cytochrome P-450. *J. Biol. Chem.* 251:1817–27.

Heilman, F. R., and Kendall, E. C. 1944. The influence of 11-dehydro-17-hydroxycorticosterone (Compound E) on the growth of a malignant tumor in the mouse. *Endocrinology.* 34:416–20.

Heston, W. E., and Andervont, H. B. 1944. Importance of genetic influence on the occurrence of mammary tumors in virgin-female mice. *J. Natl. Cancer Inst.* 4:403–7.

Hieger, I. 1930. The spectra of cancer-producing tars and oils and of related substances. *Biochem. J.* 24:505–11.

Hisaw, F. L., Velardo, J. T., and Goolsby, C. M. 1953. Competitive interaction of estrogens on uterine growth in rats. *Fed. Proc.* 12:68.

Holtkamp, D. E., Greslin, J. G., Root, C. A., and Lerner, L. J. 1960. Gonadotrophin inhibiting and anti-fecundity effects of Chloramiphene. *Proc. Soc. Exptl. Biol. Med.* 105:197–201.

Howell, J. S., Marchant, J., and Orr, J. W. 1954. The induction of ovarian tumours in mice with 9:10-dimethyl-1:2-benzanthracene. *Brit. J. Cancer* 8:635–46.

Huggins, C. B. 1930. Influence of urinary tract mucosa on the experimental formation of bone. *Proc. Soc. Exptl. Biol. Med.* 27:349–51.

Huggins, C. B. 1931. The formation of bone under the influence of the epithelium of the urinary tract. *Arch. Surg.* 22:377–408.

Huggins, C. 1954. Endocrine methods of treatment of cancer of the breast. *J. Natl. Cancer Inst.* 15:1–25.

Huggins, C. 1962. Cancer and necrosis induced selectively by hydrocarbons. In: *Horizons in Biochemistry,* edited by M. Kasha and B. Pullman, pp. 497–511. New York: Academic Press.

Huggins, C. B. 1965. Two principles in endocrine therapy of cancers: Hormone deprival and hormone interference. *Cancer Res.* 25:1163–67.

Huggins, C. 1967. Endocrine-induced regression of cancers. *Science* 156:1050–54.

Huggins, C. 1969. Epithelial osteogenesis—a biological chain reaction. *Proc. Am. Philosoph. Soc.* 113:458–63.

Huggins, C., and Bergenstal, D. M. 1951. Surgery of the adrenals. *J. Am. Med. Asso.* 147:101–6.

Huggins, C., and Bergenstal, D. M. 1952. Effect of bilateral adrenalectomy on certain human tumors, *Proc. Natl. Acad. Sci.* 38:73–76.

Huggins, C., Briziarelli, G., and Sutton, H., Jr. 1959. Rapid induction of mammary carcinoma in the rat and the influence of hormones on the tumors. *J. Exptl. Med.* 109:25–42.

Huggins, C. B., and Dao, T. L.-Y. 1952. Adrenalectomy for mammary cancer. *Ann. Surg.* 136:595–603.

Huggins, C., Deuel, T. F., and Fukunishi, R. 1963. Protection of adrenal cortex by hydrocarbons against injury from 7,12-dimethylbenz[a]anthracene. *Biochem. Ztschr.* 338:106–13.

Huggins, C., Ford, E., Fukunishi, R., and Jensen, E. V. 1964. Aromatic-induced prevention of fatal toxicity of 7,12-dimethylbenz[a]anthracene. *J. Exptl. Med.* 119:943–54.

Huggins, C. B., Ford, E., and Jensen, E. V. 1965. Carcinogenic aromatic hydrocarbons: special vulnerability of rats. *Science* 147:1153–54.

Huggins, C., and Fukunishi, R. 1963a. Cancer in the rat after single exposures to irradiation or hydrocarbons. Age and strain factors. Hormone dependence of the mammary cancers. *Radiation Res.* 20:493–503.

Huggins, C., and Fukunishi, R. 1963b. Mammary and peritoneal tumors induced by intraperitoneal administration of 7,12-

dimethylbenz[a]anthracene in newborn and adult rats. *Cancer Res.* 23:785–89.

Huggins, C., and Fukunishi, R. 1964. Induced protection of adrenal cortex against 7,12-dimethylbenz[a]anthracene. Influence of ethionine. Induction of menadione reductase. Incorporation of thymidine-H³. *J. Exptl. Med.* 119:923–42.

Huggins, C., and Grand, L. C. 1963. Sarcoma induced remotely in rats fed 3-methylcholanthrene. *Cancer Res.* 23:477–80.

Huggins, C. B., and Grand, L. 1966. Neoplasms evoked in male Sprague-Dawley rat by pulse doses of 7,12-dimethylbenz[a]anthracene. *Cancer Res.* 26:2255–58.

Huggins, C. B., Grand, L. C., and Brillantes, F. P. 1959. Critical significance of breast structure in the induction of mammary cancer in the rat. *Proc. Natl. Acad. Sci. USA* 45:1294–1300.

Huggins, C., Grand, L. C., and Brillantes, F. P. 1961. Mammary cancer induced by a single feeding of polynuclear hydrocarbons and its suppression. *Nature* 189:204–7.

Huggins, C., Grand, L., and Fukunishi, R. 1964. Aromatic influences on the yields of mammary cancers following administration of 7,12-dimethylbenz[a]anthracene. *Proc. Natl. Acad. Sci. USA* 51:737–42.

Huggins, C., Grand, L., and Oka, H. 1970. Hundred day leukemia: preferential induction in rat by pulse-doses of 7,8,12-trimethylbenz[a]anthracene. *J. Exptl. Med.* 131:321–30.

Huggins, C., and Hodges, C. V. 1941. Studies on prostatic cancer. I. Effect of castration, estrogen and androgen injection on serum phosphatases in metastatic carcinoma of prostate. *Cancer Res.* 1:293–97.

Huggins, C., and Jensen, E. V. 1954. Significance of the hydroxyl groups of steroids in promoting growth. *J. Exptl. Med.* 100:241–46.

Huggins, C., and Jensen, E. V. 1955. The depression of estrone-induced uterine growth by phenolic estrogens with oxygenated functions at positions 6 or 16: The impeded estrogens. *J. Exptl. Med.* 102:335–46.

Huggins, C., Jensen, E. V., and Cleveland, A. S. 1954. Chemical structure of steroids in relation to promotion of growth of the vagina and uterus of the hypophysectomized rat. *J. Exptl. Med.* 100:225–40.

Huggins, C., and Kuwahara, I. 1967. Effect of dexamethasone on stem-cell leukemias of rat. In: *Endogenous Factors Influencing Host-Tumor Balance,* edited by R. W. Wissler, T. L. Dao and S. Wood, Jr., pp. 9–14. Chicago: University of Chicago Press.

Huggins, C., Moon, R. C., and Morii, S. 1962. Extinction of experimental mammary cancer, I. Estradiol-17β and progesterone. *Proc. Natl. Acad. Sci. USA* 48:379–86.

Huggins, C., and Morii, S. 1961. Selective adrenal necrosis and apoplexy induced by 7,12-dimethylbenz[a]anthracene. *J. Exptl. Med.* 114:741–60.

Huggins, C., Morii, S., and Grand, L. C. 1961. Mammary cancer induced by a single dose of polynuclear aromatic hydrocarbons: Routes of administration. *Ann Surg. (Supplement)* 154:315–18.

Huggins, C. B., Morii, S., and Pataki, J. 1969. Selective destruction of adrenal cortex by pulse-doses of derivatives of 12 methylbenz[a]anthracene. *Proc. Natl. Acad. Sci. USA* 62 704–7.

Huggins, C., and Moulder, P. V. 1944. Studies on the mammary tumors of dogs. I. Lactation and the influence of ovariectomy and suprarenalectomy thereon. *J. Exptl. Med.* 80:441–54.

Huggins, C. B., and Oka, H. 1972. Regression of stem-cell erythroblastic leukemia after hypophysectomy. *Cancer Res* 32:239–42.

Huggins, C. B., Oka, H., and Fareed, G. 1972. Induction of mammary cancer in rats of Long and Evans strain. In: *Estrogen, Target Tissues and Neoplasia,* edited by T. L. Dao, pp 333–43. Chicago: University of Chicago Press.

Huggins, C. B., and Pataki, J. 1965. Aromatic azo derivatives preventing mammary cancer and adrenal injury from 7,12 dimethylbenz[a]anthracene. *Proc. Natl. Acad. Sci. USA* 53 791–96.

Huggins, C. B., Pataki, J., and Harvey, R. G. 1967. Geometry of carcinogenic polycyclic aromatic hydrocarbons. *Proc. Natl. Acad. Sci. USA* 58:2253–60.

Huggins, C. B., and Sammett, J. F. 1933. Function of the gall bladder epithelium as an osteogenic stimulus and the physiological differentiation of connective tissue. *J. Exptl. Med.* 58:393–400.

Huggins, C. B., and Sugiyama, T. 1965. Production and prevention of two distinctive kinds of destruction of adrenal cortex. *Nature* 206:1310–14.

Huggins, C. B., and Sugiyama, T. 1966. Induction of leukemia in rat by pulse-dose of 7,12-dimethylbenz[a]anthracene. *Proc. Natl. Acad. Sci. USA* 55:74–81.

Huggins, C. B., Ueda, N., and Russo, A. 1978. Azo dyes prevent hydrocarbon-induced leukemia in rat. *Proc. Natl. Acad. Sci. USA* 75:4524–27.

Huggins, C. B., and Uematsu, K. 1976. Induction of lymphatic leukemia in non-inbred mice and its control with glucocorticoids. The Lucy Wortham James Lecture. *Cancer* 37:177–80.

Huggins, C., and Yang, N. C. 1962. Induction and extinction of mammary cancer. *Science* 137:257–62.

Huggins, C. B., Yoshida, H., and Bird, C. C. 1974. Hormone-dependent stem-cell rat leukemia evoked by a series of feedings of 7,12-dimethylbenz[*a*]anthracene. *J. Natl. Cancer Inst.* 52:1301–5.

Inbar, M., and Sachs, L. 1969. Interaction of the carbohydrate-binding protein concanavalin A with normal and transformed cells. *Proc. Natl. Acad. Sci. USA* 63:1418–25.

Jellinck, P. H., Garland, M., and McRitchie, D. 1968. Effect of metopirone and 3-(1,2,3,4-tetrahydro-1-oxo-2-naphthyl)-pyridine on the metabolism of corticosteroids and DMBA in relation to adrenal necrosis. *Experientia* 24:124–25.

Jensen, E. V. 1965. Mechanisms of estrogen action in relation to carcinogenesis. *Proc. Can. Cancer Res. Conf.* 6:143–165.

Jensen, E. V., Block, G. E., Smith, S., Kyser, K., and DeSombre, E. R. 1972*a*. Estrogen receptors and hormone dependency. In: *Estrogen, Target Tissues and Neoplasia,* edited by T. L. Dao, pp. 23–57. Chicago: University of Chicago Press.

Jensen, E. V., and DeSombre, E. 1973. Estrogen-receptor interaction. *Science.* 182:126–34.

Jensen, E. V., Ford, E., and Huggins, C. B. 1963. Depressed incorporation of thymidine-H^3 into deoxyribonucleic acid following administration of 7,12-dimethylbenz[*a*]anthracene. *Proc. Natl. Acad. Sci. USA* 50:454–59.

Jensen, E. V., and Jacobson, H. I. 1960. Fate of steroid estrogens in target tissues. In: *Biological Activities of Steroids in Relation to Cancer,* edited by G. Pincus and E. P. Vollmer, pp. 161–74. New York: Academic Press.

Jensen, E. V., and Jacobson, H. I. 1962. Basic guides to the mechanism of estrogen action. *Recent Progr. Hormone Res.* 18:387–414.

Jensen, E. V., Mohla, S., Gorell, T., Tanaka, S., and DeSombre, E. R. 1972*b*. Estrophile to nucleophile in two easy steps. *J. Steroid Biochem.* 3:445–58.

Jensen, E. V., Numata, P. I., Brecher, P., and DeSombre, E. R. 1971. Hormone-receptor interaction as a guide to biochemical mechanism. In: *The Biochemistry of Steroid Hormone Action,* edited by R. M. S. Smellie, pp. 133–59. London: Academic Press.

Jensen, E. V., Suzuki, T., Kawashima, T., Stumpf, W. E., Jungblut, P. W., and DeSombre, E. R. 1968. A two step mechanism for the interaction of estradiol with rat uterus. *Proc. Natl. Acad. Sci. USA* 59:632–38.

Jungblut, P. W., Gaues, J., Hughes, A., Kallweit, E., Sierralta, W., Szendro, P., and Wagner, R. K. 1976. Activation of transcription-regulating proteins by steroids. *J. Steriod Biochem.* 7:1109–16.

Keilin, D. 1925. On cytochrome, a respiratory pigment, common to animals, yeast and higher plants. *Proc. Royal Soc. London* B 98:312–39.

Kelly, P. A., Bradley, C., Shiu, P. C., Meites, J., and Friesen, H. G. 1974. Prolactin binding to rat mammary tumor tissues. *Proc. Soc. Exptl. Biol. Med.* 146:816–19.

Kennaway, E. L. 1924. The formation of a cancer-producing substance from isoprene (2-methyl-butadiene). *J. Pathol. Bact.* 27:233–38.

Kennaway, E. L. 1930. Further experiments on cancer-producing substances. *Biochem. J.* 24:497–504.

Kidd, J. G. 1953. Regression of transplanted lymphomas induced *in vivo* by means of normal guinea pig serum. *J. Exptl. Med.* 98:565–82.

Kim, U., and Furth, J. 1960. Relation of mammary tumors to mammotropes. II. Hormone responsiveness of 3-methylcholanthrene induced mammary carcinomas. *Proc. Soc. Exptl. Biol. Med.* 103:643–45.

King, R. J. B., Cowan, D. M., and Inman, D. R. 1965. The uptake of [6,7-³H] oestradiol by dimethylbenzanthracene-induced rat mammary tumors. *J. Endocrinol.* 32:83–90.

Kinosita, R. 1936. Researches on the carcinogenesis of the various chemical substances. *Gann* 30:423–26.

Kirkman, H., and Bacon, R. L. 1950. Malignant renal tumors in male hamsters *(cricetus auratus)* treated with estrogen. *Cancer Res.* 10:122–23.

Kovacs, K., and Somogyi, A. 1969. Prevention by spironolactone of 7,12-dimethylbenz[a]anthracene-induced adrenal necrosis. *Proc. Soc. Exptl. Biol. Med.* 131:1350–52.

Kubowitz, F., and Ott, P. 1934. Isolierung und Kristallisation eines Garungsferments aus Tumoren. *Biochem. Ztschr.* 314:94–114.

Lacassagne, A. 1932. Apparition de cancers de la mamelle chez la souris mâle soumise à des injections de folliculine. *Compt. rend. Acad. Sci.* 195:630–32.

Lacassagne, A. 1937. Sarcomes lymphoïdes apparus chez des souris longuement traitées par des hormones oestrogenes. *Compt. rend. Soc. Biol.* 126:193–95.

Lacassagne, A., and Duplan, J. F. 1959. Le mécanisme de la cancérisation de la mamelle chez la Souris, considéré d'après les résultats d'experiences au moyen de la réserpine. *Compt. rend. Acad. Sci.* 249:810–12.

Lathrop, A. E. C., and Loeb, L. 1916. Further investigations on the origin of tumors in mice. III. On the part played by internal secretion in the spontaneous development of tumors. *J. Cancer Res.* 1:1–19.

Law, L. W. 1941. The induction of leukemia in mice following percutaneous application of 9,10-dimethyl-1,2-benzanthracene. *Cancer Res.* 1:564–71.

Law, L. W., and Lewisohn, M. 1940. Induction of lymphomatosis in mice following painting with 9,10-dimethyl-1:2-benzanthracene. *Proc. Soc. Exptl. Biol. Med.* 43:143–46.

Leblond, C. P., and Clermont, Y. 1952. Definition of the stages of the cycle of the seminiferous epithelium of the rat. *Ann. N. Y. Acad. Sci.* 55:548–73.

Levine, E. M. Becker, Y., Boone, C. W., and Eagle, H. 1965. Contact inhibition, macromolecular synthesis and polyribosomes in cultured human diploid fibroblasts. *Proc. Natl. Acad. Sci. USA* 53:350–56.

Lipschütz, A., Vargas, Jr. L., and Ruz, O. 1939. Antitumorigenic action of testosterone. *Lancet* 2:867–69.

Little, C. C. 1933. Existence of non-chromosomal influence in the incidence of mammary tumors in mice. *Science* 78:465–66.

Little, C. C. 1958. Biological aspects of cancer research. *J. Natl. Cancer Inst.* 20:441–64.

Little, C. C., and staff of Roscoe B. Jackson Memorial Laboratory. 1933. Existence of non-chromosomal influence in the incidence of mammary tumors in mice. *Science* 78:465–66.

Longenecker, H. E., Fricke, H. H., and King, C. G. 1940. The effect of organic compounds upon vitamin C synthesis in the rat. *J. Biol. Chem.* 135:497–510.

Lowry, O. H., Rosebrough, N. J., Farr, A. L., and Randall, R. J. 1951. Protein measurement with the folin reagent. *J. Biol. Chem.* 193:265–75.

Luft, R., and Olivecrona, H. 1953. Experiences with hypophysectomy in man. *J. Neurosurg.* 10:301–16.

Lwoff, A. 1966. Interactions entre virus, cellule et organisme.

Les Prix Nobel en 1965, pp. 233–43. Stockholm: Norstedt & Sons.

McCann, J., Choi, E., Yamasaki, E., and Ames, B. N. 1975. Detection of carcinogens as mutagens in the Salmonella microsome test: Assay of 300 chemicals. *Proc. Natl. Acad. Sci.* 72: 5135–39.

McGrath, C. M. 1971. Replication of mammary tumor virus in tumor cell cultures: Dependence on hormone-induced cellular organization. *J. Natl. Cancer Inst.* 47:455–68.

Macpherson, I., and Montagnier, L. 1964. Agar suspension culture for the selective assay of cells transformed by polyoma virus. *Virology* 23:291–94.

Macpherson, I., and Stoker, M. 1962. Polyoma transformation of hamster cell clones—an investigation of genetic factors affecting cell competence. *Virology* 16:147–51.

Maisin, J., and Coolen, M.-L. 1936. Au sujet du pouvoir cancérigène du méthyl-cholanthrène. *Compt. rend. Soc. Biol.* 123:159–60.

Maisin, J., Meerseman, F., and Maldague, P. 1956. Cancers de la mamelle chez le rat, oestrogenes et irradiation totale. *Acta Unio Intern. Contra Cancrum* 12:661–64.

Manolov, G., and Manolova, Y. 1972. Marker band in one chromosome 14 from Burkitt lymphomas. *Nature* 237:33–34.

Marchant, J. 1957. The chemical induction of ovarian tumours in mice. *Brit. J. Cancer* 11:452–64.

Mark, J. 1973 Karyotype patterns in human meningiomas. A. comparison between studies with G- and Q-banding techniques. *Hereditas* 75:213–20.

Märki, F., and Martius, C. 1960. Vitamin K-Reduktase, Darstellung und Eigenschaften. *Biochem. Z.* 333:111–35.

Martius, C., and Märki, F. 1957. Über Phyllochinon-reduktase. *Biochem. Z.* 329:450.

Mason, H. S. 1957. Mechanisms of oxygen metabolism. *Advances Enzymol.* 19:79–233.

Meister, A. 1950. Lactic dehydrogenase activity of certain tumors and normal tissues. *J. Natl. Cancer Inst.* 10:1263–71.

Meites, J. 1972a. Hypothalamic control of prolactin secretion. In: *Lactogenic Hormones, Ciba Foundation Symposium*, edited by G. E. W. Wolstenholme and J. Knight, pp. 325–38. London: Churchill Livingstone.

Meites, J. 1972b. Relation of prolactin and estrogen to mammary tumorigenesis in the rat. *J. Natl. Cancer Inst.* 48:1217–24.

Miller, E. C., and Miller, J. A. 1960. The carcinogenicity of fluoro derivatives of 10-methyl-1,2-benzanthracene. I. 3-and 4'-monofluoro derivatives. *Cancer Res.* 20:133–37.

Miller, E. C., and Miller, J. A. 1962. The induction of tumors in rats with small amounts of *N*-hydroxy-2-acetylaminofluorene or its cupric chelate. *Proc. Am. Assoc. Cancer Res.* 3:344.

Miller, E. C., Miller, J. A., and Brown, R. R. 1952. On the inhibitory action of certain polycyclic hydrocarbons on azo dye carcinogenesis. *Cancer Res.* 12:282–83.

Miller, E. C., Miller, J. A., and Hartmann, H. A. 1961. N-Hydroxy-2-acetylaminofluorene: A metabolite of 2-acetylaminofluorene with increased carcinogenic activity in the rat. *Cancer Res.* 21:815–24.

Miller, J. A., MacDonald, J. C., and Miller, E. C. 1954. The inhibition of 2-acetylaminofluorene carcinogenesis by methylcholanthrene. *Proc. Am. Assoc. Cancer Res.* 1:32.

Miller, J. A., and Miller, E. C. 1953. The carcinogenic aminoazo dyes. In: *Advances in Cancer Research*, edited by J. P. Greenstein and A. Haddow, 1:340–96. New York: Academic Press.

Miller, J. A., and Miller, E. C. 1963. The carcinogenicities of fluoro derivatives of 10-methyl-1,2-benzanthracene. II. Substitution of the K region and the 3', 6-, and 7-positions. *Cancer Res.* 23:229–39.

Mirand, E. A., and Grace, J. T. 1962. Induction of leukemia in rats with Friend virus. *Virology* 17:364–66.

Mitelman, F., and Levan, G. 1972. The chromosomes of primary 7,12-dimethylbenz[*a*]anthracene-induced rat sarcomas. *Hereditas* 71:325–34.

Mitelman, F., Mark, J., Levan, G., and Levan, A. 1972. Tumor etiology and chromosome pattern. *Science* 176:1340–41.

Mohla, S., DeSombre, E. R., and Jensen, E. V. 1972. Tissue-specific stimulation of RNA synthesis by transformed estradiol-receptor complex. *Biochem. Biophys. Res. Commun.* 46:661–67.

Monesi, V. 1962. Autoradiographic study of DNA synthesis in spermatogonia and spermatocytes of mouse testis using tritiated thymidine. *J. Cell Biol.* 14:1–18.

Monroe, J. S., and Windle, W. F. 1963. Tumors induced in primates by chicken sarcoma virus. *Science* 140:1415–16.

Montagnier, L. 1968. Corrélation entre la transformation des cellules BHK21 et leur résistance aux polysaccharides acides en milieu gélifié. *Compt. rend. Acad. Sc. Paris. D* 267:921–24.

Moon, H. D., Li, C. H., and Simpson, M. E. 1956. Effect of pituitary hormones on carcinogenesis with 9,10-dimethyl-1,2-benzanthracene in hypophysectomized rats. *Cancer Res.* 16:111–16.

Moon, H. D., Simpson, M. E., Li, C. H., and Evans, H. M. 1950. Neoplasms in rats treated with pituitary growth hormone. I. Pulmonary and lymphatic tissues. *Cancer Res.* 10:297–308.

Moon, H. D., Simpson, M. E., Li, C. H., and Evans, H. M. 1951. Neoplasms in rats treated with pituitary growth hormone. V. Absence of neoplasms in hypophysectomized rats. *Cancer Res.* 11:535–39.

Moore, C. R., and Price, D. 1932. Gonad hormone functions and the reciprocal influence between gonads and hypophysis with its bearing on the problem of sex-hormone antagonism. *Am. J. Anat.* 50:13–71.

Morgan, C. N. 1968. Surgery and surgeons in eighteenth-century London. *Ann. Royal College Surg. Eng.* 42:1–37.

Morii, S., and Huggins, C. 1962. Adrenal apoplexy induced by 7,12-dimethylbenz[a]anthracene related to corticosterone content of adrenal gland. *Endocrinology* 71:972–76.

Morton, J. J., and Mider, G. B. 1938. The production of lymphomatosis in mice of known genetic constitution. *Science* 87:327–28.

Morton, J. J., and Mider, G. B. 1941. Some effects of carcinogenic agents on mice subject to spontaneous leukosis. *Cancer Res.* 1:95–98.

Mueller, G. C., and Miller, J. A. 1949. The reductive cleavage of 4-dimethylaminoazobenzene by rat liver: The intracellular distribution of the enzyme system and its requirement for triphosphopyridine nucleotide. *J. Biol. Chem.* 180:1125–36.

Mueller, G. C., and Miller, J. A. 1953. The metabolism of methylated aminoazo dyes. I. Oxidative demethylation by rat liver homogenates. *J. Biol. Chem.* 202:579–87.

Mühlbock, O. 1956. The hormonal genesis of mammary cancer. In: *Advances in Cancer Research*, edited by J. P. Greenstein and A. Haddow, 4:371–91. New York: Academic Press.

Murphy, J. B., and Sturm, E. 1943. The adrenals and susceptibility to transplanted leukemia of rats. *Science* 98:568.

Nagasawa, H., and Meites, J. 1970. Suppression by ergocornine and iproniazid of carcinogen-induced mammary tumors in rats; effects on serum and pituitary prolactin levels. *Proc. Soc. Exptl. Biol. Med.* 135:469–72.

Nathanson, I. T. 1947. Hormonal alteration of advanced cancer of the breast. *S. Clin. North America* 27:1144–50.

Nazerian, K. 1973. Marek's disease: a neoplastic disease of chickens caused by a herpesvirus. In: *Advances in Cancer Research*, edited by G. Klein and S. Weinhouse, 17:279–315. New York: Academic Press.

Nelson, W. O. 1939. Atypical uterine growths produced by prolonged administration of estrogenic hormones. *Endocrinology* 24:50–54.

Nelson, W. O. 1944. The induction of mammary carcinoma in the rat. *Yale J. Biol. Med.* 17:217–28.

Neuhof, H. 1917. Fascia transplantation into surgical defects. *Surg. Gynec. Obstet.* 24:383–427.

Noble, R. L., and Collip, J. B. 1941. Regression of estrogen-induced mammary tumors in female rats following removal of the stimulus. *Canad. Med. Assoc. J.* 44:1–5.

Noble, R. L., and Cutts, J. H. 1959. Mammary tumors of the rat: A review. *Cancer Res.* 19:1125–39.

Nowell, P. C. 1960. Phytohemagglutinin: An initiator of mitosis in cultures of normal human leukocytes. *Cancer Res.* 20: 462–66.

Nowell, P. C., and Hungerford, D. A. 1960. Chromosome studies on normal and leukemic human leukocytes. *J. Natl. Cancer Inst.* 25:85–109.

Nowell, P. C., and Hungerford, D. A. 1961. Chromosome studies in human leukemia. II. Chronic granulocytic leukemia. *J. Natl. Cancer Inst.* 27:1013–36.

Olch, I. Y. 1937. The menopausal age in women with cancer of the breast. *Amer. J. Cancer* 30:563–66.

Oppenheimer, B. S., Oppenheimer, E. T., and Stout, A. P. 1952. Sarcomas induced in rodents by imbedding various plastic films. *Proc. Soc. Exptl. Biol. Med.* 79:366–69.

Pataki, J., and Huggins, C. B. 1969*a*. Molecular site of substituents of benz[*a*]anthracene related to carcinogenicity. *Cancer Res.* 29:506–9.

Pataki, J., and Huggins, C. B. 1969*b*. Relation of methyl and ethyl substitution of benz[*a*]anthracene to carcinogenicity. In: *Physico-Chemical Mechanisms of Carcinogenesis*, pp. 64–71. Jerusalem Symposia on Quantum Chemistry and Biochemistry. Jerusalem: Israel Academy of Sciences and Humanities.

Pazos, Jr., R., and Huggins, C. 1945. Effect of androgen on the prostate in starvation. *Endocrinology* 36:416–25.

Pearson, O. H., Eliel, L. P., Rawson, R. W., Dobriner, K., and Rhoads, C. P. 1949. ACTH- and cortisone-induced regression of lymphoid tumors in man. A preliminary report. *Cancer* 2:943–45.

Pearson, O. H., Ray, B. S., Harrold, C. C., West, C. D., Li, M. C., Maclean, J. P., and Lipsett, M. B. 1956. Hypophysectomy in treatment of advanced cancer. *J. Am. Med. Asso.* 161:17–21.

Pierpaoli, W., and Haran-Ghera, N. 1975. Prevention of induced leukaemia in mice by immunological inhibition of adenohypophysis. *Nature* 254:334–35.

Piliero, S. J. 1959. Influence of hypoxic stimuli upon blood formation in endocrine-deficient animals. *Ann. N. Y. Acad. Sci.* 77:518–42.

Pott, P. 1808. Cancer scroti. *The Chirurgical Works of Percivall Pott, F.R.S.* 3:177–83. Edited by J. Earle. London: Wood and Innes.

Prigozhina, E. L. 1962. Induction of leukosis in rats with dimethylbenzanthracene and its transplantation. *Vopr. Onkol.* 8:64–70.

Purchase, H. G. 1974. Marek's disease virus and the herpesvirus of turkeys. *Progr. Med. Virol.*, 18:178–97.

Quadri, S. K., Kledzik, G. S., and Meites, J. 1973. Effects of L-dopa and methyldopa on growth of mammary cancers in rats. *Proc. Soc. Exptl. Biol. Med.* 142:759–61.

Rauscher, F. J. 1962. A virus-induced disease of mice characterized by erythrocytopoiesis and lymphoid leukemia. *J. Natl. Cancer Inst.* 29:515–44.

Reece, R. P., and Leonard, S. L. 1941. Effect of estrogens, gonadotropins and growth hormone on mammary glands of hypophysectomized rats. *Endocrinology* 29:297–303.

Reece, R. P., Turner, C. W., and Hill, R. T. 1936. Mammary gland development in the hypophysectomized albino rat. *Proc. Soc. Exptl. Biol. Med.* 34:204–7.

Rees, E. D., and Huggins, C. 1960. Steroid influences on respiration, glycolysis and levels of pyridine nucleotide-linked dehydrogenases of experimental mammary cancers. *Cancer Res.* 20:963–71.

Rees, E. D., Majumdar, S. K., and Shuck, A. 1970. Changes in chromosomes of bone marrow after intravenous injections of 7,12-dimethylbenz[a]anthracene and related compounds. *Proc. Natl. Acad. Sci. USA* 66:1228–35.

Regaud, C., and Blanc, J. 1906. Actions des Rayons-X sur les diverses Generations de laLignee spermatique. Extrème Sensibilité des Spermatogonies a ces Rayons. *Compt. rend. Soc. biol.* 61:163–65.

Richardson, H. L., and Cunningham, L. 1951. The inhibitory action of methylcholanthrene on rats fed the azo dye 3'-methyl-4-dimethylaminoazobenzene. *Cancer Res.* 11:274.

Richardson, H. L., Stier, A. R., and Borsos-Nachtnebel, E. 1952. Liver tumor inhibition and adrenal histologic responses in rats to which 3'-methyl-4-dimethylaminoazobenzene and 20-methylcholanthrene were simultaneously administered. *Cancer Res.* 12:356–62.

Rous, P. 1911. Transmission of a malignant new growth by means of a cell-free filtrate. *J. Am. Med. Asso.* 56:198.

Rous, P. 1965. Viruses and tumour causation. An appraisal of present knowledge. *Nature* 207:457–63.

Rous, P. 1966. "Nobelpristagare I Medicin" (television interview). Sveriges Radio. Production 66/4705, November 29, 1966. B. Feldreich, producer.

Rous, P., Murphy, J. B., and Tytler, W. H. 1912. A filterable agent the cause of a second chicken-tumor, an osteochondro sarcoma. *J. Am. Med. Asso.* 59:1793–94.

Rowley, J. D. 1973. A new consistent chromosomal abnormality in chronic myelogenous leukaemia identified by quinacrine fluorescence and Giemsa staining. *Nature* 243:290–93.

Sabin, A. B., and Koch, M. A. 1963. Behaviour of noninfectious SV40 viral genome in hamster tumor cells: Induction of synthesis of infectious virus. *Proc. Natl. Acad. Sci. USA* 50:407–17.

Sanders, F. K., and Smith, J. K. 1970. Effect of collagen and acid polysaccharides on the growth of BHK/21 cells in semisolid media. *Nature* 227:513–15.

Sanford, K. K., Likely, G. D., and Earle, W. R. 1954. The development of variations in transplantability and morphology within a clone of mouse fibroblasts transformed to sarcoma-producing cells *in vitro*. *J. Natl. Cancer Inst.* 15:215–37.

Sasaki, T., and Yoshida, T. 1935. Experimentelle Erzeugung des Lebercarcinoms durch Fütterung mit o-Amidoazotoluol. *Virchow's Arch. Path. Anat.* 295:175–200.

Schubert, D., Humphreys, S., Baroni, C., and Cohn, M. 1969. *In vitro* differentiation of a mouse neuroblastoma. *Proc. Natl. Acad. Sci. USA* 64:316–23.

Schurr, P. E. 1969. Composition and preparation of experimental intravenous fat emulsions. *Cancer Res.* 29:258–60.

Schwenk, E., and Hildebrandt, F. 1932. Ein neues isomeres Follikelhormon aus Stutenharn. *Naturwissen.* 20:658–59.

Segi, M. 1960. *Cancer Mortality for Selected Sites in 24 Countries (1950–57)*. Sendai: Tohoku University School of Medicine.

Segi, M., and Kurihara, M. 1972. *Cancer Mortality for Selected Sites in 24 Countries. No. 6 (1966–1967)*. Tokyo: Japan Cancer Society.

Sharon, N., and Lis, H. 1972. Lectins: Cell-agglutinating and sugar-specific proteins. *Science* 177:949–59.

Shay, H., Aegerter, E. A., Gruenstein, M., and Komarov, S. A. 1949. Development of adenocarcinoma of the breast in Wistar rat following the gastric instillation of methylcholanthrene. *J. Natl. Cancer Inst.* 10:255–66.

Shay, H., Gruenstein, M., Marx, H. E., and Glazer, L. 1951. The development of lymphatic and myelogenous leukemia in Wistar rats following gastric instillation of methylcholanthrene. *Cancer Res.* 11:29–34.

Shay, H., Harris, C., and Gruenstein, M. 1952. Influence of sex hormones on the incidence and form of tumors produced in male or female rats by gastric instillation of methylcholanthrene. *J. Natl. Cancer Inst.* 13:307–31.

Shear, M. J., and Leiter, J. 1940. Studies in carcinogenesis. XIV. 3-Substituted and 10-substituted derivatives of 1,2-benzanthracene. *J. Natl. Cancer Inst.* 1:303–36.

Shellabarger, C. J., Cronkite, E. P., Bond, V. P., and Lippincott, S. W. 1957. The occurrence of mammary tumors in the rat after sublethal whole-body irradiation. *Radiation Res.* 6:501–12.

Shope, R. E. 1933. Infectious papillomatosis of rabbits. *J. Exptl. Med.* 58:607–24.

Sinha, D., Cooper, D., and Dao, T. L. 1973. The nature of estrogen and prolactin effect on mammary tumorigenesis. *Cancer Res.* 33:411–14.

Staff of the Jackson Memorial Laboratory. 1933. The existence of non-chromosomal influence in the incidence of mammary tumors in mice. *Science* 78:464–65.

Stich, H. F. 1960. Chromosomes of tumor cells. I. Murine leukemias induced by one or two injections of 7,12-dimethylbenz[a]anthracene. *J. Natl. Cancer Inst.* 25:649–61.

Stoker, M. G. P. 1972. Tumour viruses and the sociology of fibroblasts. *Proc. Royal Soc. London B* 181:1–17.

Stoker, M., O'Neill, C., Berryman, S., and Waxman, V. 1968. Anchorage and growth regulation in normal and virus-transformed cells. *Int. J. Cancer* 3:683–93.

Sugiyama, T. 1971a. Role of erythropoietin in 7,12-dimethylbenz[a]anthracene induction of acute chromosome aberration and leukemia in the rat. *Proc. Natl. Acad. Sci. USA* 68: 2761–64.

Sugiyama, T. 1971b. Specific vulnerability of the largest telocentric chromosome of rat bone marrow cells to 7,12-dimethylbenz[a]anthracene. *J. Natl. Cancer Inst.* 41:1267–75.

Sugiyama, T. 1973. Capillary hematocrit method combined with microscopical observation and its application to a quick screening of rat leukemia. *Acta Path. Japan* 23:1–9.

Sugiyama, T., Kurita, Y., and Nishizuka, Y. 1967. Chromosome abnormality in rat leukemia induced by 7,12-dimethylbenz-[a]anthracene. *Science* 158:1058–59.

Sutherland, E. W. 1972. Studies on the mechanism of hormone action. Nobel Lecture. In: *Les Prix Nobel en 1971*, pp. 240–57. Stockholm: Norstedt & Sons.

Sydnor, K. L., Butenandt, O., Brillantes, F. P., and Huggins, C. B. 1962. Race-strain factor related to hydrocarbon-induced mammary cancer in rats. *J. Natl. Cancer Inst.* 29:805–14.

Sydnor, K. L., and Cockrell, B. 1963. Influence of estradiol-17β, progesterone and hydrocortisone on 3-methylcholanthrene-induced mammary cancer in intact and ovariectomized Sprague-Dawley rats. *Endocrinology* 73:427–32.

Szent-Györgyi, A., Isenberg, I., and Baird, Jr., S. L. 1960. On the electron donating properties of carcinogens. *Proc. Natl. Acad. Sci. USA* 46:1444–49.

Talalay, P., Takano, G. M. V., and Huggins, C. 1952. Studies on the Walker tumor. II. Effects of adrenalectomy and hypophysectomy on tumor growth in tube-fed rats. *Cancer Res.* 12:838–43.

Temin, H. M., and Mitzutani, S. 1970. RNA-dependent DNA polymerase in virions of Rous Sarcoma Virus. *Nature* 226: 1211–13.

Todaro, G. J., and Green, H. 1963. Quantitative studies of the growth of mouse embryo cells in culture and their development into established lines. *J. Cell Biol.* 17:299–313.

Toft, D., and Gorski, J. 1966. A receptor molecule for estrogens: isolation from the rat uterus and preliminary characterization. *Proc. Natl. Acad. Sci. USA* 55:1574–81.

Touster, O., Hester, R. W., and Siler, R. A. 1960. The inhibition by ethionine of the enhancement of ascorbic acid excretion by barbital and 3-methylcholanthrene in the rat. *Biochem. Biophys. Res. Comm.* 3:248–52.

Turner, F. C. 1941. Sarcoma at sites of subcutaneously implanted bakelite disks in rats. *J. Natl. Cancer Inst.* 2:81–83.

Udenfriend, S., Clark, C. T., Axelrod, J., and Brodie, B. B. 1954. Ascorbic acid in aromatic hydroxylation. I. A model system for aromatic hydroxylation. *J. Biol. Chem.* 208:731–39.

Uematsu, K., and Huggins, C. 1968. Induction of leukemia and ovarian tumors in mice by pulse-doses of polycyclic aromatic hydrocarbons. *Mol. Pharmacol.* 4:427–34.

Uematsu, K., and Huggins, C. 1969. Hydrocarbon-induced leukemia in adolescent and adult mice. *Gann* 60:545–55.

Van Dyke, D. C., Contopoulos, A. N., Williams, B. S., Simpson, M. E., Lawrence, J. H., and Evans, H. M. 1954. Hormonal factors influencing erythropoiesis. *Acta Hematol.* 11:203–22.

Warburg, O. 1910. Ueber die Oxydationen in lebenden Zellen nach Versuchen am Seeigel-Ei. *Z. Physiol. Chem.* 66:305–30.

Warburg, O. 1930. *The Metabolism of Tumours*, translated by F. Dickens. London: Constable & Co.

Warburg, O. 1948*a*. *Schwermetalle als Wirkungsgruppen von Fermenten*. Berlin: Verlag Dr. Werner Saenger.

Warburg, O. 1948*b*. *Wasserstoffubertragende Fermente*. Berlin: Dr. Werner Saenger.

Warburg, O. 1969. *The Prime Cause and Prevention of Cancer*, translated by D. Burk. Würzburg: K. Triltsch.

Warburg, O., Gawehn, K., and Geissler, A.-W. 1958. Ueber die Entstehung des Krebsstoffwechsels in der Gewebekultur. *Z. Naturforsch.* 13B:61–63.

Warburg, O., Posener, K., and Negelein, E. 1924. Ueber den Stoffwechsel der Carcinomzelle. *Biochem. Ztschr.* 152:310–44.

Ward, H. W. C. 1973. Anti-oestrogen therapy for breast cancer: A trial of Tamoxifen at two dose levels. *Brit. Med. J.* 1:13–14.

Waterhouse, R. 1911. A case of suprarenal apoplexy. *Lancet* I:577–78.

Wattenberg, L. W., and Leong, J. L. 1965. Effects of phenothiazines on protective systems against polycyclic hydrocarbons. *Cancer Res.* 25:365–70.

Wattenberg, L. W., Leong, J. L., and Strand, P. J. 1962. Benzpyrene hydroxylase activity in the gastrointestinal tract. *Cancer Res.* 22:1120–25.

Weber, G. 1961. Behaviour of liver enzymes during hepatocarcinogenesis. In: *Advances in Cancer Research*, edited by A.

Haddow and S. Weinhouse, 6:403–94. New York: Academic Press.

Weber, G. 1968. Carbohydrate metabolism in cancer cells and the molecular correlation concept. *Naturwissen.* 55:418–29.

Weber, G. 1974. The molecular correlation concept: Recent advances and implications. In: *The Molecular Biology of Cancer,* edited by H. Busch, pp. 487–521. New York: Academic Press.

Welsch, C. W. 1972. Effect of brain lesions on mammary tumorigenesis. In: *Estrogen Target Tissues and Neoplasia,* edited by T. L. Dao, pp. 317–31. Chicago: University of Chicago Press.

Wheatley, D. N., Hamilton, A. G., Currie, A. R., Boyland, E., and Sims, P. 1966. Adrenal necrosis induced by 7-hydroxy-methyl-12-methylbenz[a]anthracene and its prevention. *Nature* 211:1311–12.

Wieland, H., and Dane, E. 1933. Untersuchungen über die Konstitution der Gallensäuren. LII. Über die haftstelle der Seitenkette. *Z. Physiol. Chem.* 219:240–44.

Williams-Ashman, H. G., and Huggins, C. 1961. Oxidation of reduced pyridine nucleotides in mammary gland and adipose tissue following treatment with polynuclear hydrocarbons. *Med. Exper.* 4:223–26.

Wilson, R. H., DeEds, F., and Cox, Jr., A. J. 1941. The toxicity and carcinogenic activity of 2-acetaminofluorene. *Cancer Res.* 1:595–608.

Wintrobe, M. M. 1933. Macroscopic examination of the blood. *Am. J. Med. Sci.* 185:58–71.

Woolley, G., Fekete, E., and Little, C. C. 1939. Mammary tumor development in mice ovariectomized at birth. *Proc. Natl. Acad. Sci. USA* 25:277–79.

Woolley, G. W., and Little, C. C. 1945a. The incidence of adrenal cortical carcinoma in gonadectomized female mice of the extreme dilution strain. I. Observations on the adrenal cortex. *Cancer Res.* 5:193–202.

Woolley, G. W., and Little, C. C. 1945b. The incidence of adrenal cortical carcinoma in gonadectomized female mice of the extreme dilution strain. III. Observations on the adrenal glands and accessory sex organs in mice 13 to 24 months of age. *Cancer Res.* 5:321–27.

Woolley, G. W., and Little, C. C. 1946. Prevention of adrenal cortical carcinoma by diethylstilbestrol. *Proc. Natl. Acad. Sci. USA* 51:737–42.

Yamagiwa, K., and Ichikawa, K. 1916. Experimentelle Studie

über die Pathogenese der Epithelialgeschwűlste. mitt Fakultät K. Japanisches Universität Tokyo. 15:295–344.

Yamagiwa, K., and Ichikawa, K. 1918. Experimental study of the pathogenesis of carcinoma. *J. Cancer Res.* 3:1–29.

Yang, N. C., Castro, A. J., Lewis, M., and Wong, T. W. 1961. Polynuclear aromatic hydrocarbons, steroids and carcinogenesis. *Science* 134:386–87.

Yang, S. K., and Dower, W. V. 1975. Metabolic pathways of 7,12-dimethylbenz[a]anthracene in hepatic microsomes. *Proc. Natl. Acad. Sci. USA* 72:2601–5.

Young, S. 1961. Induction of mammary carcinoma in hypophysectomized rats treated with 3-methylcholanthrene, estradiol-17β, progesterone and growth hormone. *Nature* (London) 190:356–57.

Zilber, L. A., Lapin, B. A., and Adgighytov, F. I. 1965. Pathogenicity of Rous sarcoma virus for monkeys. *Nature* 205:1123–24.

Zondek, B., and Bergmann, E. 1938. Phenol methyl ethers as oestrogenic agents. *Biochem. J.* 32:641–45.

Zymbal, W. E. 1933. Histologische und experimentelle Untersuchungen am Epithelgewebe der Talgdrüsen (Gehörgangdrüse der Ratte). *Z. Zellforsch. mikr. Anat.* 18:596–625.

Index